"I wish I'd known earlier..."

Ten things about fertility that could change your life

'I WISH I'D KNOWN EARLIER …'

TEN THINGS ABOUT FERTILITY THAT COULD CHANGE YOUR LIFE

Anne Hope

BSc (Hons) PGCE LCCH RSHom

Claire Chaubert

BSc (Hons) LCCH RSHom RM

Published in 2015 by Telos Publishing Ltd

5A Church Road, Shortlands, Bromley, Kent BR2 0HP, UK

'I Wish I'd Known Earlier …': Ten Things About Fertility That Could Change Your Life © 2015 Anne Hope and Claire Chaubert

Design: Mark Stammers

ISBN: 978-1-84583-910-9

British Library Cataloguing in Publication Data. A catalogue record for this book is available from the British Library.

Disclaimer

This book is for information and education purposes only. It is not intended to and does not offer individual medical advice or diagnosis to any reader.

AUTHORS' NOTE

The individual experiences recounted in this book are drawn from actual clients we have seen in our clinic. However, the names and potentially identifying details have been changed to protect their identities and confidentiality.

We work from a clinic in South London. If you would like further information please visit our website at www.homeopathyfertilityclinic.com

With thanks to Gia D'Aprano for her research work.

Anne Hope and Claire Chaubert

January 2015

CONTENTS

Introduction   9

1. The Starting Point -
Understanding Your Cycle!   15

2. PCOS (Polycystic Ovarian Syndrome) –
'My cycles have come back and
the cysts disappeared.'   23

3. The AMH (Anti-Mullerian Hormone) Debate –
'My eggs are old, they say nothing can be done.'   31

4. A High Level of Natural Killer Cells –
Could this be the reason I'm not pregnant?'   39

5. Sperm Quality Can Be Changed   49

6. Is Unexplained Infertility Really Unexplained?   61

**7. 'Things aren't quite how they used to be after
contraception/first baby/ trauma/grief ...'**   67

8. Emotions and Stress – 'Do these really
make a difference?'   83

9. IVF – 'Can anything improve my chances
of IVF working?'   103

10. Early Miscarriage/Repeated Miscarriage –
'Is this ever going work?'   113

A Final Word   121

Bibliography   123

About the Authors   127

INTRODUCTION

For over ten years now, we have been running a specialist fertility clinic in which we have used homeopathic and other natural methods to treat dozens of women and their partners who have come to us with a range of fertility-related problems. In this book, drawing on the extensive knowledge and experience we have gained, we aim to shed light on ten of the most common issues about fertility that have been raised with us.

Our clinic is, we believe, unique in its approach. However, by using a series of anonymised real-life case studies, we will explain our observations, understanding and results in a clear, straightforward way that we hope will offer help and encouragement to anyone facing such problems, and show that there are often positive steps that can be taken and options available.

~~~~~~

CASE STUDY – NADIA

'We had been trying for a baby for two years with no success, two years of trying all the old wives' tales – ice baths, legs in the air etc etc – and although this was fun (!) we just couldn't hit the jackpot! We seriously tried not to get stressed, went on lots of holidays, tried not to think about it and probably ended up trying too hard.

'So, two years later, we decided to seek professional help; a long and slow process. After seeing our GP we

were referred to an NHS consultant and had the usual battery of tests, only to be told that we had "unexplained infertility". So, onto the IVF rollercoaster, and we had two costly failed attempts at this, only to be told we had less than 5% chance of IVF working.

' "Enough," we said of all this. Five years and nothing – there had to be something else. My husband said "Let's try homeopathy." "What a hippie," I thought! Coming from a medical background, I had little faith and lots of scepticism, but just thought, "Well why not?", as my husband had used it before with complete success.

'We saw Claire and Anne, who listened encouragingly, and suddenly we were made to feel like human beings with a problem to sort out that wasn't insurmountable. At last a proactive stance!

'So after two hours we walked out with a plan and lots of funny plastic bags with little white pills, and dutifully took them. "Could this really work?" I thought, while my husband did nothing but offer positivity.

'A month later, we were back, with our charts filled in, with Claire and Anne smiling with encouragement. Going on holiday from that appointment, we went armed with the little pills. "Hmm …" A week later, when we came home, my period was a week overdue. Now that was strange. "I'm going to do a pregnancy test," I said, and before the two minutes were up, there, appearing faintly, was the second line …

'My little girl was born in November 2009, and we are going to try for another baby soon.'

The case above is a simple one but in many ways typifies accounts given by our satisfied clients. The vast majority of them initially have no belief or faith in homeopathy, but come to us as a 'last chance' when everything else has failed. They have no answers, nowhere else to turn. But by carefully going over the individual case history, we can usually see a way forward. With over 3,500 homeopathic remedies available, we have a choice of treatments, and have developed a way of combining these to work as quickly and efficiently as possible.

Clients will sit in front of us and explain their 'intractable' problem. Most have been told there is nothing further that can be done to change their situation. Some have been told that the only solution is high levels of medication – which either haven't work or are causing negative side effects. Some have even been offered major surgery – which may not actually solve the problem, but is the best idea their doctors have been able to come up with at that moment.

We have seen women suffering very heavy periods offered a hysterectomy as the only solution when medication fails – but in some cases these are young women who might well want a family someday. These clients come to us feeling let down, depressed, frustrated, angry and ultimately out of control. When we explain to them that their problem is probably a result of hormonal imbalances that can be fixed, it changes everything.

Sometimes couples have been many years down the road of trying for a baby, with all the associated relationship pressures – which can cause difficulties between themselves, with their wider families, with friends who have had babies, or with work colleagues who may all seem to be complaining about their children. For someone with fertility problems, having a friend or a colleague who is pregnant – and dealing with all the natural but often guilty emotions this prompts, such as envy, anger and grief – so often becomes deeply self-destructive.

When the long process of doctors, referrals, tests, even investigatory surgery, has led nowhere, and the doctors say they don't really know, what then?

We feel that people deserve to have choices, and to know that alongside the medical model there are other effective ways of helping with both male and female infertility and with problem cycles.

The feedback we typically get from clients is that they feel anger that pursuing a conventional medical solution has needlessly wasted so much of their valuable time and money, along with the accompanying emotional investment. In our society, doctors seem to have the final say on people's prognosis – but often our clients come to us with a very poor prognosis, and this changes during the course of treatment. Having encountered problems they had believed permanent and immovable – polycystic ovarian syndrome (PCOS), low anti-mullerian hormone (AMH), etc – they find they now have a possible explanation and solution, and often say things like, 'I only wish I'd known earlier …', 'People deserve to know …', 'You should write a book …'

Well, this is that book.

Homeopathy, and how we work

To put the material in the following chapters into context, we ought to start by explaining a little about homeopathy, and about how we work in our clinic.

Every cell of the body has a DNA mapping of how it is supposed to function. The body thus has an inherent ability and predisposition to heal itself. For example, a broken leg, once set straight, will successfully rebuild bone tissue, nerve fibres, muscles, skin etc. This is an amazingly complex natural phenomenon, which we can take for granted. Despite the body having what we know is a natural ability to heal itself, we sometimes doubt its capacity to address certain problems, believing that a conventional medical approach is the only possibility for regaining health. When the body changes, and doesn't work as it should, it can become stuck in a cycle of increasing dysfunction.

Homeopathy aims to trigger the body's underlying healing capacity, essentially pushing a 'reset button' so that it can go back to its original and correct way of working. It is a safe and gentle method based upon the principle of like curing like – so that any substance that can make you ill can also, in homeopathic form, treat you. Its effectiveness has been demonstrated empirically over more than two hundred years – it is the world's second most used system of medicine – as well as in a number of independent trials. Treatment is highly individualised, and remedies – usually administered in the form of small white pills – are made from a huge variety of materials including minerals, plants and animal sources.

The very fine balances of hormones that control so many aspects of our lives, such as stress levels, depression, anger and happiness, also control our reproductive ability. They feed back to each other, and one being slightly out of balance can gradually cause a whole cycle imbalance. In our clinic, we work by taking a complete case history of the individual, including their medical history, stresses, worries and concerns. We use a system of prescribing that we have found to be not only effective, but as fast and efficient as possible at correcting problems. The remedies all work together to target areas we feel are out of balance. These are both physical and mental/ emotional. The body works as a whole, so it is important to treat the person as a whole.

1   THE STARTING POINT – UNDERSTANDING YOUR CYCLE!

It is surprising and shocking that many women haven't been taught to understand the implications of how their cycle functions. This is true even of some women who have undergone lengthy medical interventions and medications, and it leaves them unable to make a realistic assessment of the success of their treatment.

We are taught that a healthy or good cycle is usually regular, 28-30 days, that ovulation happens around day 14, and that if menstruation (bleeding) occurs for about 3-5 days, it can be assumed all is well.

This is far from the whole story.

The noticeable signs of the menstrual cycle (bleeding/ovulation) are only a demonstration or reflection of the hormonal changes and shifts that are happening throughout the whole of a woman's fertile years. The cycle is extremely subtle, and each hormone forms part of a wider feedback system.

There are a number of different hormones at work, and what a woman may observe through her cycle is the interaction of these complicated sweeps. These hormones must all be in balance and proportionate to each other in order for a cycle to be truly healthy.

When we see clients, we are looking for signs and symptoms of this balance and how it may have changed for them over the years. From our observations, it appears that many women don't really recognise that this is particular and individual to them. It is rare that we have a whole day in our clinic without encountering one of the common misunderstandings addressed below. In fact, the misunderstandings are almost mythological; people believe that if they observe certain characteristics about their cycle, then all is well. As with many myths, there is an element of truth in them, but we need to look at them in context.

Cycle length myth

'I have a normal 28 day cycle, so why aren't I getting pregnant?'

Although 28 days is the 'classic' figure, there is a normal variation in timing and length of cycle. Text books don't always take account of this. We examine every part of a client's cycle, and often find that a 'classic'-length cycle is not actually natural or normal for that particular woman. A cycle needs to be of optimum length for that individual in order for it to be genuinely fertile. Homeopathy is ideal for creating this natural balance. The remedies can stimulate the body to allow the cycle to be of the correct length, the bleed to be appropriate, and ovulation to take place at the right time for each individual.

Ovulation timing myth

'I ovulate on day 14, like I'm supposed to, so why aren't I getting pregnant?'

The optimum time to ovulate is 14 days before bleed. On a

'classic' 28-day cycle this is also, coincidentally, midpoint. So common misunderstandings have arisen that a woman should:

- ovulate 14 days after bleed, irrespective of cycle length; and/or

- ovulate mid-cycle, whatever the individual cycle length (e.g. ovulate on day 17 of a 34-day cycle).

CASE STUDY – TAMI

'I came to see Anne and Claire, having been trying to get pregnant for three years without success. I had had some basic hormone tests, which showed I probably wasn't ovulating. The doctors offered me Clomid to get me to ovulate, but I wasn't happy to take it. I've never done very well on hormonal medication such as the pill; it's always made me feel terrible.

'Anne and Claire talked through my cycle with me in much more detail than I ever had before – I even had to send my husband out of the room! I realised that I might be ovulating later than I thought. I thought that everyone who had a 28-day cycle ovulated on day 14. When I did ovulation tests all through my cycle, I discovered I was actually ovulating on day 21, and Claire explained to me that the cycle length should be longer. Only seven days after ovulation was too little time for the hormones to build to hold a pregnancy.

'After six months of treatment, my cycle settled at 35 days, and I ovulated on day 21 every month.

'I thought that my cycle had to be 28 days long, and I realise now that the doctors' attempts to adjust it to that length were making everything worse.

'Now I have two lovely children.'

Ovulation myths

'If I am bleeding I must be ovulating, surely?'

'I am not bleeding. Does that mean I'm not ovulating?'

'The ovulation tests come up negative. Does this mean I'm not ovulating?'

Over-the-counter ovulation tests are only about 80% effective at predicting ovulation, although some are a little more sensitive than others. This means that about one in five times they won't give an accurate result. They work differently from home pregnancy tests, which test for a particular hormone that the body releases if there is a pregnancy and are very accurate. Ovulation tests test for any hormones excreted in the urine, rather than for just a particular 'ovulation hormone'.

While there are more accurate tests available, these are blood tests that your doctor would need to organise for you. These give better indications about whether or not ovulation is likely to have occurred, as they analyse which specific hormones were present when the bloods were taken.

Some women don't use ovulation tests. They assume that because they are bleeding, this means they must have ovulated. However, you can bleed without ovulating, because some of the hormones may build a lining in the first half of your cycle, but their levels may still be insufficient to develop a healthy, fully mature egg.

Conversely, although it is more unusual to ovulate without a bleed, this is possible, and we have seen this in a number of clients. Pregnancy in this case can be more difficult to achieve, as it does indicate a hormonal imbalance that needs to be rectified.

Balance

Balance is the key word, and shots of drugs to artificially induce ovulation or bleed are at best crude tools. Very similar prescriptions are given by doctors to all women with this problem, regardless of the degree of imbalance. In some cases this approach does work – the drugs and treatment are sufficient and successful. It is therefore understandable that for clinicians this would appear to be a sensible first step. At our clinic, however, we see people for whom this approach has not been successful or has made them feel worse. When medical treatment hasn't worked, people often feel without any alternative except simply to repeat that treatment. Even when the first, second or even fifth IVF treatment hasn't succeeded, some couples feel there is no option but to keep trying the same thing.

This is where the alternative, holistic approach we take

is so positive, as our clients realise that, even though drugs haven't been successful for them, they aren't at the end of the road, and more choices are available to them. Many of them come to see us with their systems in a more imbalanced state following drug intervention than they were before they sought medical treatment – there can be almost a see-saw or pendulum effect, where the cycle becomes ever more dysfunctional as the body tries to compensate for the additional stimulus. While one aspect of the cycle may look better, with apparent improvements such as mid-cycle ovulation, we still see many cases where this has not led to the goal of successful pregnancy.

Not everyone who seeks homeopathic treatment has gone down the conventional medical route first. Sometime people want to try a non-drug-based system as a primarily approach to improve their fertility. They are not necessarily against medication, but feel that a more holistic and individualised methodology is the best option for them.

Inducing ovulation isn't necessarily the sole goal. The quality of the egg and the underlying hormones that support it are also critical to achieving a successful pregnancy. It is heart-breaking when the hormones are insufficiently balanced, as this will prevent a successful conception and subsequent pregnancy developing. We have seen women suffering repeated early miscarriages, and their cycles fluctuating due to the body no longer having proper control over the very delicate changes needed to conceive and carry a child.

CASE STUDY – CHERYL

'I had been trying to get pregnant for two years, so I went to the doctor, who sent me for loads of tests. They couldn't really see what was wrong, so eventually I ended up having IVF. I took all the different injections and kept to their plan, but had an awful reaction to the drugs – I thought it was just normal for IVF, but I actually had ovarian hyper-stimulation syndrome, which made me feel terrible and meant that I had to stop the treatment. To be honest, my cycle was never back to normal again, and it just seemed to be a bit haywire. We were so desperate to have a baby that we just went straight back in for another IVF cycle, and I hyper-stimulated again. I couldn't face more IVF after that and didn't know what to do. A friend recommended Claire and Anne – I had no idea what homeopathy even was, but was desperate, nothing could make anything worse.

'After my first appointment I realised my cycle was way out, and it didn't seem like it was going back by itself. Thankfully, once I started treatment, I saw things returning to normal; in fact much better than before I started IVF, more how it was when I was teenager. Although I'm only three months into treatment, I now have a strong ovulation and a good bleed. I now don't have PMT, and for the first time in a long time I am hopeful for the future.'

Having a really good understanding of your own cycle and what is natural and normal for you is a really essential part of your health and wellbeing. As homeopaths, we talk our clients through all of these details and enable them to understand where the issues may lie, what we need to target, and how we will aim to change and restore their natural hormonal cycles.

2 PCOS (POLYCYSTIC OVARIAN SYNDROME) – 'MY CYCLES HAVE COME BACK AND THE CYSTS DISAPPEARED.'

Polycystic ovarian syndrome (PCOS) is one of the most common causes of female infertility, and of hormonal problems in young women generally. It produces symptoms in approximately 5% to 10% of women of reproductive age.

The symptoms and their severity vary greatly between women, but are often distressing and/or embarrassing. The most common immediate symptoms are irregular menstruation (bleeding), no menstruation, lack of ovulation, acne and excessively oily skin. Some more severe cases also present with excess hair and/or hair in inappropriate places such as nipples, chest, back and face. It is common in these cases to have weight gain that is almost impossible to shift. As well as all these physical symptoms, women with PCOS may feel poorly, or unbalanced emotionally and mentally.

All of these symptoms are due only to a hormonal imbalance – albeit a very complex one – that produces cysts on the ovary instead of effective ovulations. Although medication may alleviate some of the symptoms, it is not curative. Unsurprisingly, therefore, we see a lot of clients with this condition. Some are actively trying to get pregnant, while others just want to get rid of the PCOS. They want to feel well and to have their body working properly.

To date, all of the dozens of cases of PCOS we have treated homeopathically have resulted in full clearance of cysts, as confirmed by ultrasound scans. This is not just a reduction of symptoms, or even a temporary lessening of visible cysts, but is a long-lasting change. Scans taken even some years later have shown no cysts returning, and women's cycles still being strong, healthy and normal.

This is a bold statement and runs counter to the perceived wisdom that PCOS is incurable and will only get more severe over time. However, it is worth reiterating that the women we see are generally those for whom conventional treatment hasn't worked – some individuals do find medication sufficient to contain their symptoms.

CASE STUDY – EMILY

'I had already done lots to help my PCOS. I'd done a lot of research and followed strict nutritional advice, taken lots of good-quality supplements, had exercise sessions with a personal trainer four times a week. I knew it was an uphill battle – lots of women in my family have serious PCOS, and I didn't want to be the fat, hairy stereotype!

'This really did help my weight and "hairiness", but I still had no periods, no ovulation at all, and still had cysts that showed up on every scan – although I have to say they weren't growing as fast as the doctors thought they might do with my family history (especially as I didn't want to take metformin).

'I wanted to have children at some point, and thought I should look at this before it became a block. After a year of treatment at the homeopathic clinic, at their suggestion I had a scan, because my periods were back to normal. I wanted to know if it had made any inroads on the cysts themselves. I was thrilled, but the doctors were shocked, when they saw I was completely clear of cysts.

'It has now been three years since my initial treatment, and a recent scan has shown I still have no cysts at all on my ovaries.'

PCOS in detail

The most typical hormone changes associated with PCOS are raised levels in the blood of male hormone (testosterone) and luteinising hormone (LH), and insulin resistance. The simplest explanation for the syndrome is that the ovary makes an excess of testosterone by one of two mechanisms:

1. **The ovary might be overactive in its testosterone production, spontaneously releasing testosterone without the corresponding and balancing hormones; or**

2. **The ovary might be driven to produce excess testosterone by the action of either LH or insulin.**

Insulin resistance is associated with obesity, high cholesterol levels and type two diabetes. (However, to be clear, PCOS does not necessarily lead to diabetes – as mentioned above, the severity of the syndrome varies between women.) Insulin is a hormone responsible for keeping the blood sugar levels in normal range. If blood sugar is out of balance, this means that insulin is not being produced or used appropriately. Therefore regulating blood sugar and insulin can be useful in managing some of the symptoms of PCOS.

Conventional medical treatment

The only drug currently available in the UK that reliably reduces insulin concentrations is metformin. This is an indirect treatment for PCOS, which addresses the insulin/testosterone balance. It attempts to reduce testosterone levels, reduce cyst growth and make the menstrual cycle more regular. This can be useful in slowing growth or holding things as they are, and the lessening of symptoms can help some women, particularly if the PCOS is mild. However, it fails to resolve the underlying hormonal imbalance that is at the heart not only of PCOS but of many infertility problems. If the patient stops taking the metformin, the symptoms will usually return.

Women who are having difficulty becoming pregnant and have been diagnosed with PCOS may also be given a drug, usually clomiphene, intended to stimulate ovulation. Again, in some cases, particularly where the PCOS is mild, this can be sufficient. However, the clients we see have usually already attempted the available medical treatments without success. Using drug treatments such as clomiphene stimulates one aspect of the system without addressing the underlying problem.

If your goal is to have a baby and/or to be medication-free, then resolving the underlying problem is best.

Diet can really help

Studies have shown that a good low glycaemic index diet, together with high-quality targeted supplements, can correct insulin imbalance. The glycaemic index (GI) of foods is a ranking of how they affect blood sugar levels. Slowly-absorbed foods have a low GI rating, and those that are absorbed rapidly and cause spikes in blood sugar levels have a high GI rating. So choosing foods that have a low GI enables smooth and balanced blood sugar levels throughout the day.

Examples of foods to avoid (high GI):

- simple sugars, bananas, dried fruits, fruit juices;
- refined carbohydrates such as white rice, white bread and pasta;
- saturated fats and trans fats;
- sugary and carbonated drinks.

Examples of foods to eat (low GI):

- vegetables, lentils and pulses;
- complex carbohydrates such as buckwheat, rye, quinoa;
- wholemeal bread;
- nuts and seeds;
- lean protein such as chicken.

Homeopathic treatment

Not all PCOS cases are the same. Some women we see have no cycles at all and no underlying signs or symptoms of any active hormones (e.g. pre-menstrual tension (PMT), bloating, mood swings etc). Others have irregular or occasional bleeds, perhaps only one every three to four months, or extended light bleeding with a lot of spotting, all of which can indicate unbalanced or ineffective hormones. Strangely, some women can experience very heavy, erratic periods as well.

Our homeopathic treatment is individualised, and we have to take into account the different presentations to determine the appropriate remedies to tackle the problems. There is no simple, single solution. We may wish to tackle the cysts themselves, getting the body to reabsorb them. On other occasions we may wish to address the lack of bleeding or the development of endometrium (i.e. mucous membrane lining the inside of the uterus). In every instance we are looking to restore a balanced hormonal cycle.

Both men and women have what are typically thought of as male and female hormones. In healthy, fertile women there is a preponderance of oestrogen and a low level of testosterone. Women with PCOS have an imbalance of these hormones, and a higher level of testosterone than is ideal or supportive of a healthy, fertile cycle.

There is no need to think of PCOS as a life sentence. As stated above, every client we have treated for this syndrome is now free of it. The human body has a natural tendency to wish to return to health, and homeopathic remedies aim to support the body to resolve the inappropriate hormone levels.

Many people have said they wished they had known earlier that PCOS can be changed.

THE AMH (ANTI-MULLERIAN HORMONE) DEBATE – 'MY EGGS ARE OLD, THEY SAY NOTHING CAN BE DONE.'

In the last few years, the AMH test has proved a popular one among doctors seeking to treat fertility problems. It is a blood test to check the level of a particular hormone, known as the anti-mullerian hormone, and is done between day two and day five in the cycle – often on day three. The blood test is analysed and a figure is given that is then interpreted as being good, normal or low. The standard interpretation of this test is that a decreased level or low level of AMH may signify a low ovarian reserve, i.e. there are too few eggs left in the ovaries or the eggs are old, indicating diminishing fertility.

Woman are often told that a low level of AMH may indicate premature ovarian failure, or minimal or reduced responsiveness to IVF treatment, meaning that their chances of natural conception are reduced to almost nil. This is typically used to explain why conception has not taken place – especially if a couple have been trying unsuccessfully for some considerable time.

Many couples who come to our clinic have been led to believe that its levels are fixed. The AMH reflects the age of the eggs, they have been told, and therefore the quality; and like our general physical ageing, the ageing of the eggs cannot be reversed. The only solution for poor AMH, they have been advised, is egg donation. These couples, some of whom have been trying for a pregnancy for years, are understandably shocked to have been given this news, which feels like a devastating and final blow.

Contrary to this received medical wisdom, we have found that the AMH result is not fixed. It can and does improve and change following expert homeopathic treatment – as demonstrated when the test is repeated and reflects the now-fertile state of the woman's eggs. Women with previously poor AMH levels have conceived both naturally and through IVF following our treatment, which has improved their hormonal cycle.

This new test result would seem to indicate that the eggs have got younger – which orthodox opinion would say is impossible! In fact, the use of the word 'age' in relation to the eggs is misleading. Unlike a person's physical age – something that only ever increases – the 'age' of the egg is actually a measure of how it is growing and maturing throughout the woman's cycle. So a poor 'age' for an egg would indicate that there is a problem with the cycle and how it is maturing the egg at that particular point in time. Improving the cycle changes the egg's 'age' and accordingly the AMH level.

Scientific research backs this up. [1] AMH levels can vary between menstrual cycles and within one cycle alone. This in itself demonstrates that the AMH test is testing something more than the egg reserve, i.e. the number of eggs left.

If you are in or near menopause, the eggs will not be maturing very well at all – this will be reflected in the AMH being measured as low, as there is little effective maturation occurring. Therefore it is true that menopause or near menopause will

---

[1] *Loh and Makeshuari (2011), cited in Clarke et al (2014), Human Reproduction Volume 29(1) pp 184-187).*

give a low AMH result. This is a natural reflection of the ending of the fertile period in a woman's life. However, it is not always true that low AMH equals the onset of menopause. It does mean low quality eggs, which can have a variety of causes, the most common of which we see being sluggish ovulation. When our homeopathic remedies are used to improve ovulation, the AMH readings change and improve, creating a more fertile cycle.

CASE STUDY – LAURA

'When the fertility doctors told us that our eggs were old, I was shocked. I was only 28, and had been trying to get pregnant since I got married two years earlier. I had expected normal blood tests and perhaps IVF treatment – but they told me that it was like my eggs were 45 years old, and that my only realistic chance of being a mum was egg donation.

'I'm not sure they realised how devastating and unexpected this was. I just thought that I'd have to take some medication and it would sort things out. I had no problem with that. This felt like a whole other ball game. I just didn't know what to do.

'A friend recommended the homeopathic fertility clinic, but it was down in London, and I lived several hundred miles away. But when I found out that consultations could be done by Skype, I thought I'd give it a shot – there seemed nothing to lose.

'It did seem like a slow start initially, and I wasn't sure if much was happening. My periods seemed a little

better, but no big deal. When I asked how long the process would take, Claire and Anne said to leave it three to six months and then get retested. I went back to the hospital after five months, and really expected nothing to have changed. I was gobsmacked when the results of the tests showed that the age of my eggs matched my real age – I wasn't an old lady anymore!'

The science and the debate

In one research study, PCOS patients were tested for AMH levels.[2] These were shown to give a false measurement of poor ovarian reserve. Women with PCOS are known to have low quality or ineffective egg maturation, and yet even here the levels of AMH were not fixed but subject to daily fluctuations. The whole notion of exactly what is being tested by measuring AMH levels is not clear, and researchers have highlighted problems with testing protocols between the various laboratories. They have also shown how vulnerable the tests are to technical errors that can provide false measurements.

Overall the scientific community itself questions the utility and reliability of the AMH test as a definitive biomarker of the health of egg-producing follicles within the ovary. There is, as yet, no standardisation of measurement.

The medical profession's current tendency to view low AMH test results as the principal cause of infertility fails to take

[2] *Hadlow et al 2013 ibid – in Clarke 2014.*

into account other factors that can affect the production of the hormone. Couples may even be refused IVF treatment on the basis of a low AMH result.

Other factors that affect AMH include certain hormones (gonadotropins), lifestyle stresses, past use of the contraceptive pill, and thyroid and autoimmune conditions.

What low AMH really shows us

It is true that when we treat couples who have been diagnosed with low AMH, the woman's menstrual cycles often reflect poor egg quality. However, the range of variables that contribute to poor egg quality, some of which are outlined above, requires a holistic approach to address the problem.

CASE STUDY – SUSAN

'I wasn't really surprised but was upset to hear that my ovarian reserve test showed my eggs were old – I was 43. But I didn't expect the reaction and treatment I got from the doctor. I was effectively told that I was stupid thinking I could get pregnant. He actually laughed, and I felt like I wanted the ground to open up under me.

'But then I got angry and decided not to take what I'd been told. A colleague seemed to have had a "lucky" result with the homeopathy fertility clinic, so I had a go too – it could hardly make things worse. What really

*surprised me was that, after treatment, my periods
changed, I had positive ovulation tests, I felt emotionally
completely changed, even my libido came back! I felt back
in charge of my life and hormones again.'*

In this client's case, there was no ovulation most of the time, and when it did occur it was too late in the cycle. This meant that the AMH reading was simply reflecting a poor egg maturation, which made the egg appear 'older' than in fact it was.

Some researchers feel it is inadvisable to attribute diagnostic or prognostic significance to an AMH value as a stand-alone measure of ovarian reserve.[3] It certainly appears to indicate hormonal imbalance resulting in poor maturation of the egg. This should give hope to couples who in the past believed the 'sentence' of low AMH levels meant they had little chance of conceiving – AMH levels are not only subject to variation, they can be improved upon!

In order to understand how this is achievable, it is useful to understand a little of the egg maturation process itself. Eggs take three of the woman's cycles to mature fully. Each of those three cycles has to have exactly the right hormones released at exactly the right time. The egg needs to ovulate at exactly the right time as well – 12 to 24 hours too late can be fatal for the 'ripeness' of the egg. So if the hormones are sluggish, it is likely to take too long to mature the egg.

Think of a sponge cake cooked on too low a heat. It takes a lot longer and will certainly not be light and spongy when

---

[3] *Clarke et al 2014.*

eventually taken out of the oven! It will be overcooked; but taking it out earlier would have meant it was underdone. This is a simple analogy of how things have to be just right to produce the right results.

Just because the egg quality looks 'old' at the time of an AMH test, in our experience this doesn't mean the eggs really are necessarily old. By giving homeopathic remedies that target specific hormones over a two to three month period, we seek to change the long-term egg maturation process and improve egg quality.

The stem cell debate

It is an accepted wisdom that women are born with a set number of eggs that eventually 'run out'. Many a time a client has said to us, 'My AMH is low, I have only a few eggs left.' A recent research study[4] has suggested that instead of having a finite number of eggs that run out, women are instead born with stem cells in their ovaries that have the ability continually to produce new eggs as needed.

This research has called into question the idea that the small pool of germ stem cells in the ovaries actually contributes to the production of immature follicles with the potential to produce new eggs. Nevertheless, such studies have generated interest in creating new experimental hormonal treatments to target stem cell activity in adult female ovaries.

Caution should of course be exercised in using any such new and unproven treatments where no conclusive evidence is

---

[4] *Bhartiya et al 2013.*

available. The key point is that preliminary research results can be easily turned into a generic proclamation of women's fertility potential, before the full ramifications of the research work have been properly assessed.

Homeopathy can make its contribution by providing individualised treatment regimes that take into account the specific person and situation. By using a raft of deep-acting remedies that stimulate the complex and interconnected hormonal systems orchestrating all the various facets of infertility, we have successfully counteracted the poor prognosis for many couples.

4 A HIGH LEVEL OF NATURAL KILLER CELLS – 'COULD THIS BE THE REASON I'M NOT PREGNANT?'

Over the years we have been running our homeopathy fertility clinic, we have seen come and go a succession of fashions and fads, whereby some simplistic new idea or other has been seized upon by the medical profession to 'explain' infertility. These fads always seem to coincide with a new strand of research – and research funding – related to an expensive new form of treatment being developed by pharmaceutical companies.

All of a sudden, couple after couple will start turning up at our clinic saying they have been told that they might have a certain newly-identified condition, which is not backed up by scientific research but could be a reason why 'things' aren't happening. These couples, who are often desperate and looking for answers, are naturally inclined to seize upon any such explanation, however thinly supported it might be. The fact that they have not been offered any remedial treatment, or worse still have been offered very expensive treatment that has not been shown to be effective, then brings heartache.

The real heartache for us is the misinformation – perhaps inadvertent – that is so often taken as fact by the couples. They contact us with what they have been told is a diagnosis giving them no way out of their condition, when this may be far from the truth.

One recent fad seems to concern natural killer cells, which – it is claimed – may prevent a fertilised egg from implanting in the uterus. In fact, the science does not support a high level of natural killer cells being a common condition responsible for infertility. Although we have come across two rare cases where it might be the cause, in every other instance where a client has come to see us with this diagnosis, it has turned out, after examination of their case and homeopathic treatment, that they don't actually appear to have this problem.

Both of the women we have seen who genuinely had a high level of natural killer cells had extremely robust immune systems. They never got colds, sore throats, tummy bugs or other common infections, and hadn't done even as a child.

CASE STUDY – CARLA

'Being only 26, I expected to get pregnant easily. After it not happening for a year, we had a bit of a panic, and were sent off for some basic tests, which all seemed fine. There had to be a reason, so we went private, and they suggested another test, because they thought my immune system was too strong and rejecting the pregnancy. When the test showed that this might be the case – the doctor said it was on the high side – it seemed to make sense to me. They were the experts, after all.

'They suggested steroids, so I had IVF with these and a few other drugs that they said were especially good for this condition. I was so hopeful. They seemed to know what they doing. Each time, they changed what I took, but it always made me feel awful, without any positive result.'

After speaking to this client we felt it unlikely that natural killer cells were playing any role in her fertility problems. She had a normal frequency of typical ailments such as coughs, colds, sore throats, viruses – not indicative of an overly active immune system. The diagnosis our client had been given had effectively sent her down a cul-de-sac, as not only is the relevant blood test – known as the Chicago test – scientifically controversial, in that it may not accurately reflect what is really going on in the uterus, but there is no effective treatment for a high level of natural killer cells.

Natural killer cells are needed by the body. They are a normal and healthy part of our immune system and necessary for our survival. When a woman becomes pregnant, there is a natural lowering of the immune system in order to accept and develop a fertilised egg – which contains 50% of genes that are from the father and are therefore by definition alien to the mother. 'Common sense' therefore suggests that anything that threatens to stop the immune system becoming weaker at this time may prevent a conception happening or a pregnancy continuing. If a woman has too high a level of natural killer cells, surely this will kill sperm off as they enter her body, or else stop an egg with a foreign sperm in it from developing … well won't it?

Not necessarily.

It is always dangerous to correlate facts in this way. For instance, only one in six road traffic accidents is caused by a drunk driver, so five out of six occur when the drivers are perfectly sober – but it would be incorrect to conclude from this that if I want to get home safely, my best bet is to find a drunk driver to take me! Simply linking two pieces of information together does not necessarily reveal a meaningful connection – there has to be causation, i.e. one thing causes the other.

Does the level of natural killer cells in a woman's blood have any relation to the hormonal changes that allow the toleration of a 'foreign body' in the form of a developing foetus? Let's look at what is really known.

A high level of natural killer cells may not necessarily reduce your chances of conception

A healthy immune system response involves white blood cells, also known as lymphocytes, neutralising pathogens that are identified as foreign invaders in the body. About 5% of these lymphocytes are natural killer cells, and on routine contact with other cells they will actively dispense with any that do not carry a protein identifying them as belonging to that person's own body. They will also effectively deal with any body cells that have been infected with viruses, bacteria or cancerous growths.

It had been postulated that such cells might be responsible for repeated miscarriages, until it was discovered that the uterus has its own version of natural killer cells present in large numbers at implantation and early pregnancy. These uterine natural killer cells are believed to be instrumental in facilitating the linkages between the placenta and the mother's blood supply.[5] They remain in the endometrium – the lining of the uterus – and do not enter the general circulation.

So we can see that the level of natural killer cells in the blood does not necessarily bear any relation to that in the uterus. Although conventional fertility clinics have made much

---

[5] *Human Fertility and Embryology Authority, 2010.*

of the presence of high levels of natural killer cells in blood samples, given that there is no conclusive evidence of these causing repeated miscarriages, it seems unlikely that testing for them yields any useful information about the uterine environment.[6]

The level of a woman's natural killer cells varies considerably according to the stage of the menstrual cycle, with a measurement of anything up to 12% in peripheral blood samples considered normal. So, even leaving aside the fact that the level of natural killer cells in the blood tells us nothing about the level in the uterus, it seems incredible that a high detected level can be cited as the possible cause of unexplained infertility.

Conventional medical treatment

The medical profession tend to regard high levels of natural killer cells as a form of autoimmune condition. Couples may find doctors offering them costly treatments involving high-dose steroids (routinely used in the treatment of arthritis, asthma and other autoimmune disorders), intravenous immunoglobulin, and tumour necrosis factor-alpha (TNF) blocking agents. As made clear by the Human Fertilisation and Embryology Authority, none of these treatments is licensed for use, and all carry both risks and serious side effects that – as doctors often tell their patients – are considered out of proportion to their benefits. And this is all without any convincing evidence base to support those supposed benefits.

---

[6] *Moffett et al (2004) 'Natural Killer Cells, Miscarriage and Infertility'. British Medical Journal Volume 329 (7477) pp 1283-1285.*

Taking each of the treatments in turn:

Corticosteroids – These are designed to suppress the immune response and have a long history of use in the treatment of autoimmune diseases such as multiple sclerosis, rheumatoid arthritis, etc. Using them in early pregnancy has no proven advantage. On the contrary, as discussed in more detail below, some new studies suggest the possibility that using steroids may be linked to an increased risk of miscarriage. The lining of the womb, the endometrium, is known to have high levels of its own natural killer cells – particularly at the implantation site. These actually increase in pregnancy right up to 20 weeks' gestation. The use of steroids in early pregnancy is linked to an increased risk of high blood pressure, diabetes and premature birth.[7]

Intravenous immunoglobulin (IVIg) – This is produced from the blood plasma of many different donors and again is normally used to treat immune deficiencies. It shouldn't be taken lightly; it is, after all, a blood product and carries risks that can be unpredictable and severe. Side-effects range from the relatively minor, such as headache, muscle pain and general malaise, to the major, such as kidney failure and anaphylaxis. As with all blood products, there is a risk of contracting donor infections and viruses such as Creutzfeldt-Jakob disease (CJD) and hepatitis. The IVIg by its very nature contains antibodies that do cross to the developing baby.

TNF – The body's natural reaction to any form of damage or a foreign body is to create what is called an inflammatory response. This is a complex process, flooding the affected area with blood and white cells to tackle the problem. TNF

---

[7] *Rai et al (2005) 'Natural Killer Cells and Reproductive Failure – Theory, Practice And Prejudice.' Human Reproduction 20 (5) p1123-1126.*

blocks this ability of the body, including the natural killer cells, to mount an inflammatory response. The theory is that by stopping the natural killer cells creating an immune response, the body will not reject a pregnancy. However, there are major known risks to TNF drugs and a very real concern about their experimental nature. None of them is licensed to be used in pregnancy. Their makers warn that they may increase the risk of suffering septicaemia; tuberculosis; lymphatic cancer; and liver problems.

In short, all of these treatments are experimental; there is no clear evidence to suggest they help in any way to improve fertility; and their risks can be major. They are very invasive, very expensive and the side effects are not really well known. And of course alongside all these drawbacks are the fear and worry that couples face on being told that they have an insurmountable problem. All in response to a measurement that is, at best, misleading; as mentioned above, the blood test for natural killer cells doesn't relate to those found in the uterus in any event.

Homeopathic treatment

Most clients who come to the homeopathy fertility clinic having been diagnosed with a high level of natural killer cells as a 'red flag' have been given the impression by their doctors that there is very little that can be done to improve matters. Our usual first reaction in such cases is to look more broadly, and not just focus on the immune system. There is a natural process of hormones changing and supporting appropriate levels of natural killer cells in the uterus; and, as mentioned above, these cells change throughout the cycle and with pregnancy. We tend to treat people constitutionally; that is, to help strengthen and support their natural balance, rather than target this as a problem.

Men have natural killer cells too

High levels of natural killer cells have also been diagnosed as a possible cause of infertility amongst men, as they may well reduce the quantity of viable sperm. One of the most well-reported effects of a reversed vasectomy is natural killer cells attacking sperm now considered as foreign to the body and as targets for elimination! This is an observed phenomenon.

In such cases, we use our homeopathic remedies to try to increase sperm production and improve their performance. The invasive surgical procedure of the reversed vasectomy has changed the natural balance of how natural killer cells work in this instance; but we can help weight the war, giving the sperm a better chance of survival. Although natural killer cells still attack the sperm, we have found that in some cases couples have become pregnant naturally following our treatment, while in others the man has produced better quality sperm and they have been more successful with IVF. This is, however, a more difficult problem to address, as there has been an invasive procedure changing the way the body works, rather than an imbalance caused by other factors.

Steroids and miscarriage

As recently as 2008, the prevailing medical advice was to avoid taking steroids during pregnancy. Since then it has become almost routine for couples undergoing IVF at some clinics to have steroids prescribed as part of the drug protocol. This again appears to be based on the presumption that successful pregnancies need a lowered immune system – steroids suppress your immune system, the reasoning goes, therefore steroids must be good for pregnancy. It is worth remembering here the analogy of the safe driver being the drunk driver!

All of this appears to suggest that the link between the general immune system, natural killer cells in the blood and uterine immune suppression is more complicated than previously thought. Certainly it appears to be hormonally driven and to work rather differently from the anti-disease system our bodies use to protect against germs and viruses.

The Scientific Advisory Committee of the Royal College of Obstetricians and Gynaecologists (RCOG) has published a recent opinion paper on the subject of treatment of high levels of natural killer cells and other immune-system based treatment.[8] This paper states, 'Measurement of peripheral blood natural killer (PBNK) cell numbers or activity as a surrogate marker of events at the maternal-foetal interface is inappropriate … A recent large UK study reported [using] PBNK cell levels in predicting IVF cycle outcome to be "little better than tossing a coin".' In essence this means that the level of natural killer cells in the uterus provides no real measure of the chances of success or lack of success in achieving pregnancy.

The paper concludes: 'With the exception of aPL [anti-phospholipid antibodies] testing among women with recurrent miscarriage, there is little evidence to support any particular

---

[8] *Regan et al (2011) 'The Investigation and Treatment of Couples with Recurrent First-Trimester and Second-Trimester Miscarriage.' Green Top Guidelines 17 RCOG pp 1-18.*

test or immunomodulatory treatment in the investigation and treatment of couples with reproductive failure. These tests and treatments should be restricted to those entered into formal research studies.'

Further research in this area

Readers might like to be aware that the British Fertility Society (BFS) have also published a review of evidence for use of medical adjuncts (supplementary procedures) in IVF, which covers a range of immunological tests and treatments:

> L Nardo et al (2009) 'Medical adjuncts in IVF: evidence for clinical practice.' *Human Fertility* 12 (1): 1-13.

Two papers reviewing the science of NK cells in pregnancy are freely available:

> Moffett A, Regan L, Braude P. 'Natural Killer Cells, Miscarriage and Infertility.' *British Medical Journal*. 2004; 329: 1283-1285.

> Rai R, Sacks G, Trew G. 'Natural Killer Cells And Reproductive Failure – Theory, Practice and Prejudice.' *Human Reproduction*. 2005; 20(5): 1123-1126.

In summary

If natural killer cells have been mentioned to you by your doctor – don't despair! There may well be another perspective and answers other than 'There is nothing that can be done.'

5 SPERM QUALITY CAN BE CHANGED

A couple visited our consulting room a few months ago for their first appointment with us. As usual they were polite but obviously doing their best to cover their scepticism of homeopathy – although they were willing to 'give it a go'. This lack of confidence was compounded by the fact that the man's sperm results were poor. He began by telling us, 'I know there's nothing you can do to help me – the doctor told me that the sperm would have always been like this – so we've really come to see if you can make my partner feel a bit less stressed.'

The doctor's diagnosis was compounded by the fact that this man had done all the normal things that are supposed to improve sperm production: a good diet; exercise; no alcohol or smoking; etc. Once he had followed these steps, really there was no more the medical profession could do but count the sperm presented and inform him of the results. Because there are no drugs or conventional treatments available for the condition, doctors will say there is nothing that can be done. This couple, like so many others, had been told that ICSI (intra-cytoplasmic sperm injection) or sperm donation were their only options.

The couple were amazed when we explained that there was a lot we could do through homeopathic treatment to help improve sperm. We give remedies that aim to tackle poor morphology, forward motility, low volume and high viscosity – which are the common problems with sperm. We recommend a client retakes a sperm test four to six months after beginning treatment, although test results should improve after three months. This retesting will clearly show whether or not there has been any improvement in these areas. A very high proportion of our clients do show improved test results.

The technique of IVF and ICSI has its limitations – it is an intense form of treatment that works for only approximately 35% of patients. A fuller description of IVF and ICSI is given in Chapter 9, but essentially IVF involves using drugs to stimulate the ovaries, collecting the eggs and then combining them with sperm. Where the sperm is considered poor quality, then ICSI may be recommended – in these cases, a sperm is selected that looks the best in the sample, the tail of the sperm is removed and the sperm is injected into the egg. The fertilised egg is then returned to the woman's uterus, often after a number of days to observe growth and cell division in the fertilised egg. The couple must then wait to see if this successfully implants.

For the couple in the case study below, this process was problematic; it hadn't worked previously and the woman didn't do very well on the IVF drug protocol. However, considering the alternative of sperm donation was not something they were comfortable with.

CASE STUDY – CHRIS

'We came to see Claire and Anne as I really believed in alternative treatment and had been incensed when doctors had told me we had no hope of a natural conception, and that even ICSI might not work for us. My last three sperm tests had shown only two or three

individual sperm existed – not even measured as a percentage!

'I was surprised when Claire and Anne realised that my partner had some problems with her cycle too, which it seemed on reflection would have caused problems with IVF working anyway. The doctors, once they had found my problem, had just asked my partner if she had periods, and when she said yes, they hadn't investigated any further.

'I threw myself into the homeopathic treatment, as well as following all the diet advice, taking supplements and even having acupuncture. My partner was given remedies too, and we were amazed when her cycle changed and became a little shorter with a stronger bleed.

'Five months after starting treatment I had another sperm test, which came back normal! Two months later, my partner became pregnant naturally, and we now have a lovely little boy.'

What can I do to improve sperm health?

Simple approaches that are relatively well known are beneficial and can make a real difference, so shouldn't be disregarded. They may not be the complete answer, and we do find couples who get unnecessarily stressed about 'breaking rules' by having the odd wrong thing in their diet or the occasional alcoholic drink. As we will explain further in this book, stress is much more harmful than the odd glass of wine! Relaxing has a really positive effect on the body. However, it is worth bearing in mind the following tips:

- Eat a good diet with plenty of fruit and vegetables; these are rich in natural antioxidants. There is good evidence that these act as important means of mopping up the potentially damaging by-products of normal body chemistry that can otherwise act to damage developing sperm.[9]

- Keep fit and have a healthy weight; some research suggests that obesity negatively affects sperm quality, reducing sperm count and movement.

- Keep scrotal temperature relatively low; it should be a couple of degrees below body temperature.

- Avoid tight underwear or clothing.

- If you sit for long periods of time, take frequent breaks.

- Avoid smoking, which can reduce sperm count, movement and morphology. Marijuana has a major impact on sperm; the sperm actually swim in circles!

- Alcohol can affect quality and quantity of sperm, so avoid drinking too much.

- Lubricants can often contain substances that act as spermicide, so be careful which you use – natural oils are better, and pro-seed lubricant will not affect sperm.

- Forgive yourself if you fall 'off the wagon'; it is important to manage stress!

[9] Agarwal et al 2008.

Following these suggestions is a really good approach to maintain the health of sperm that are already pretty much okay to good. It is called a maintenance approach. A good analogy is that you need a certain amount of vitamin C in your diet to avoid scurvy, and a certain amount of vitamin D to avoid rickets; the Government quantifies this amount as the RDA, or recommended daily allowance.

So on a maintenance level, keeping the scrotum cool (for instance) will help prevent good sperm becoming poor. However, on a therapeutic level, keeping the scrotum cool will not make poor sperm become good. The same is true of all the above suggestions.

If you are trying to correct a problem using vitamins, you need therapeutic levels of them. These levels are way beyond the RDAs, and more than can be gained from a normal healthy diet. Not only do the levels need to be higher, but the vitamins need to be in a form that can be well used by the body. This means that they need to be really good food-state vitamins – ones that the body can fully absorb and use as if they were food. Most vitamins that can be bought in pills over the counter have a chemically-made structure that merely resembles the structure of food-state vitamins. The body can tell the difference and, depending on the quality of the product, can sometimes lose more from breaking down and eliminating this foreign substance than it gains from it.

The make and quality of vitamin pills really do matter. In our clinic, we give clients specific advice about such pills – including quantity and quality – depending on the problem presented, and the vitamins work in conjunction with homeopathic remedies to help the body reabsorb hormones.

It is the reabsorption of hormones, not just the production of them, that allows the body to make full use of them, helping to create the building blocks of correct hormonal function.

What does the sperm test really tell us?

After a semen sample is given, an initial visual inspection is made. This gives few markers to indicate whether or not the sperm is of sufficient quality, so a more detailed analysis is then carried out.

The World Health Organisation (WHO) guidelines on what constitutes good quality semen were revised at the end of 1999 and took account of extensive studies on the semen of 4,500 men in 14 different countries spread over four continents. All these men had their fertility confirmed through their partners becoming pregnant and having a live birth within less than a year of trying to conceive.

The typical volume of semen collected in a sample is around a half to one teaspoonful (two to six millilitres) of fluid. Less semen indicates fewer total sperm, which would affect fertility. More semen indicates too much fluid, which would dilute the concentration of sperm, also impeding fertility. The semen should initially be thick and then become thinner within 10 to 30 minutes. If this does not occur, it may reduce sperm movement.

Sperm concentration (also called sperm density) is measured in millions of sperm per millilitre of semen. The normal count is 20 million sperm or more per millilitre, with more than 80 million sperm in one ejaculation. Fewer sperm and/or a lower sperm concentration may reduce fertility and therefore the chances of pregnancy.

The percentage of moving sperm in a sample is known as its 'motility'. The rate and direction of travel of the sperm are also assessed. At least 50% of sperm should be motile one hour after ejaculation, and they should be moving forward in a straight line with good speed. The progression of the sperm is rated from zero to four, with a rating of three to four indicating good motility. If less than half the sperm are motile, a stain is used to identify dead sperm. This is called a 'sperm viability test'.

Another type of analysis, called 'morphology analysis', looks at the size, shape and appearance of the sperm cells. It evaluates the structure of 200 sperm, with any defects being noted. The more abnormal sperm that are present, the lower the likelihood of fertility.

Semen pH (a measure of acidity versus alkalinity) should normally be between 7.2 and 7.8, and the fructose level between 150 and 600 milligrams per decilitre (mg/dL), and there should be fewer than 2,000 white cells per millilitre.

So these figures from the WHO guidelines give us a baseline against which to assess other men – but what is often overlooked is the fact that if a man's semen results fall below these figures, that does not necessarily mean that he is infertile. As noted earlier, the guidelines are based on averaging out the results of a large number of men who have had their fertility proved. If your sperm count is lower than the guideline figure, for instance, that does not mean it is impossible to conceive; it may well reduce your chances, but this is a largely unknown area.

Doctors will usually recommend ICSI or IVF, as that is the only option they have for increasing the chances of successful pregnancy. One thing clients often say to us is, 'My sperm quality isn't really important, because doctors are going to use ICSI anyway.' Actually, though, we have found this isn't the full story.

Does sperm quality matter when ICSI is an option?

As mentioned, ICSI involves cutting the tail off a sperm and injecting it directly into an egg in order to fertilise it. The fertilised egg (embryo) is then transferred to the woman's womb. This procedure can mean that as long as some sperm can be obtained (even in very low numbers), fertilisation may be possible.

Success rates for ICSI range from a high of 35% for those under the age of 35 to a low of 5% for those of 44 years. Considering how much of the element of chance this treatment takes out of the process of conception, these rates appear to be very low. This must mean that there is more than just the ability of the sperm to swim, meet and fertilise the egg that has an impact on successful pregnancy. The statistics suggest that age is a factor, and the medical profession would explain the lack of success in older couples by saying that sperm and egg quality deteriorate as age increases. The quality of the initial cell mass that leads to the development of the embryo relates to the quality of the individual egg and sperm.

Medical assessment of the quality of the individual sperm really consists of just a visual inspection – a more rigorous assessment can be carried out only by using an analysis that pulls apart the sperm and consequently destroys that sperm sample! In truth, this is an art as well as a science. However, after taking our homeopathic remedies, men generally find that their sperm test results improve. This means that even if ICSI is, for some reason, still the preferred option, there may be more sperm to choose from; and in some cases where ICSI hasn't worked before, it has subsequently been successful.

Allowing an egg and sperm to come together naturally allows for natural selection to take place, and this may be one reason why artificial fertilisation is less successful. This supports the idea that if anything can be done to improve the overall sperm quality before the ISCI embryologists make their selection, this will improve the chances of successful pregnancy. In providing treatment it is important to consider both partners, so that the woman's hormonal cycle and egg are optimised and the sperm quality and quantity are addressed. We have found that following treatment with us, and improved sperm tests, there have often been positive results.

DNA fragmentation testing

All cells of the body naturally break down and are renewed. This cell break down/cell death (apostosis) releases sections or fragments of DNA that can be tested for. A sperm DNA fragmentation test is not routinely done by fertility doctors but can give very important further information about poor sperm test results and may be worth considering, particularly if there is a history of recurrent miscarriage or repeated unsuccessful assisted fertility treatment.

If a test shows that sperm DNA fragmentation levels are high (typically considered as over 30% of sample showing evidence of this) it demonstrates that the sperm cells are prone to an unusually high level of mutation and breakdown. Such sperm are far less likely to lead to a successful, full term pregnancy. Simply put, the subsequent fertilised egg/embryo is just not as good.

Such a poor result can feel like a body blow, but there are actually a number of possible causes – many of which can be improved upon and changed. As with other aspects of male infertility, poor sperm quality due to high levels of DNA fragmentation can respond well to a treatment programme that includes dietary antioxidant supplementation (including high quality vitamin C, vitamin E , Coenzyme Q10 etc) and selected key remedies that aim to address sperm formation and how the body metabolises hormones and nutrients.[10]

Sperm test results can be improved

Sperm take about 70 days to mature – so from the start of treatment we allow about four to six weeks for our remedies to change the sperm, then 70 days for the maturation. Sometimes however effects are apparent more rapidly. About half the men we see notice that their ejaculate has visible differences quite quickly. Most report that it is thinner (the most common problem is that semen that is too thick) and that there is more of it, and occasionally they report that the ejaculation is more powerful. These clients also generally remark that they now remember this is what it used to be like when they were younger!

---

[10] *Tarozzi et al 2007.*

Changes to sperm often occur slowly over many years, and relatively minor changes can become more entrenched and lead to greater levels of dysfunction and hormonal imbalance. While adopting a healthy diet, avoiding cigarettes and alcohol are helpful, we have found that these steps are not enough by themselves to address the poor quality of sperm our clients often report.

We tackle the problem on several levels: we address the hormonal cycles responsible for sperm; provide advice on supplements and antioxidants; suggest lifestyle changes; select remedies to reduce stress (which is known to disorder the production of hormones needed for healthy sperm); and also look for specific areas of concern – poor motility, morphology, calcium build up in the testes, etc.

With our unique approach, we target homeopathic treatment at these areas to help sperm production reach its optimum. Sperm quality can be changed; and we have many cases of empirical evidence to demonstrate that this is possible.

6   IS UNEXPLAINED INFERTILITY REALLY UNEXPLAINED?

We live in a culture where having a diagnostic label for a health issue is expected – even if the condition does not have treatment options or a solution available. For many people, having a label can feel helpful, at least initially. It is what most people expect to get when seeing a doctor.

So, it can be especially devastating for those for whom there is evidently a problem when they are told it is 'unexplained'. As one of our clients revealed to us:

'We felt cast adrift. Nobody knew what was wrong, and apparently nothing could be done that hadn't already been tried. We felt desperate and a lost cause. Even if they could say it was due to "something", at least we would know. Somehow if we thought if it was understandable then it might be easier to accept.'

Typically when people come to see us they have already gone through a battery of exploratory procedures. These normally start with a simple blood test for the woman on day 21 of her cycle, which gives a base level of information about her hormones – particularly progesterone and follicular stimulating hormone (FSH) – from which the clinician will infer whether or not ovulation is likely to have taken place. An ultrasound scan may be carried out to determine if there are any obvious growths, and a laparoscopy/dye test is often recommended. This involves inserting a small probe camera through the abdomen and also through the vagina into the uterus to look for any problems in the uterus, ovaries or abdomen or any blockages/scarring in the fallopian tubes. These tests can be useful in ruling out problems such as damaged fallopian tubes, which would prevent a successful conception.

Having been subjected to all these tests and often more, the woman and her partner will often be told that the results are all clear and within normal range. The next stage may be for the woman to be given a drug that stimulates ovulation, even where the tests have already shown that this does not appear to be the problem. The doctors will then generally recommend an IVF treatment, despite it being unclear whether or not the initial conception is the problem. Many couples then go on to have IVF and ICSI, again with no success.

Unexplained infertility remains one of the leading and growing reasons for clients to seek our help. These couples are devastated and lost. There is no reason identified for their failure to conceive, so what can anybody do?

Well, the truth is, we can do a lot. In the vast majority of cases, we have found clear and evident reasons for the infertility; but these are problems for which there is no standard medical diagnosis or treatment. The advice from these couples' doctor should not therefore be that there is nothing that can be done, but that there is nothing *they* can do!

When we see couples, we discuss and consider full details of the woman's menstrual cycles – now and in the past - and her medical and personal history, in order to determine where the issues lie. Frequently the menstrual cycles are found to be unbalanced.

The cause of the lack of balance or dysfunction can be varied, including the effect of hormonal contraceptives; the fact that the woman has never been well since a previous pregnancy or birth; previous birth trauma; or profound grief or stress. It is important to consider all of these factors and fully treat and support women and their partners, not simply address physical symptoms.

We take a very detailed look at every aspect of their hormonal cycles, and are also keen to see the results of any medical tests they may have had done. There may not be a single identifiable problem, but there may be a number of small, interrelated issues. These issues individually would not lead to infertility, but taken together can cause the system to become dysfunctional.

There may be proportionality issues. Even if tests show that hormones are 'within normal range', they may still not be right for that particular individual, or may be disproportionate to each other, with one at the high end of the normal range and others at the very bottom. The body functions best when hormones are in proportion to each other. A good, everyday analogy is height: the average woman may be between 5' 3" and 5' 8", and the average inside leg may measure from 26" to 34", but it would be very strange and disproportionate to have a 5' 8" tall woman with a 26" inside leg!

Another common problem is thyroid function. All hormones interact with each other, and we have observed how important thyroid function is to the key fertility hormones and overall fertility. Many women present with a history of underactive thyroid and are consequently taking levothyroxine – an artificial drug source of thyroxine – to supplement this. While the medication can improve the blood test results, this does not necessarily mean that the absorption of the thyroxine is ideal, and women for whom this is the case commonly experience low energy, sluggish/slow cycles that are not genuinely fertile and weight gain despite a good diet.

Using homeopathic remedies and specialist supplements, we work to address both the production of thyroxine by the thyroid and the absorption of this important hormone. This can enable women to begin discussing with their doctors reducing or even gradually eliminating the drugs they are taking.

Couples who come in with the diagnosis of unexplained infertility often have a whole range of negative emotions that can form a really toxic mix. They can feel inadequate, guilty, angry, jealous and desperate. They can be full of fear about the future. Because they have been given effectively a 'non-diagnosis', this leaves them feeling very uncertain and not knowing whether they should feel hopeful or give up.

The effect on the relationship between the couple can be profoundly destructive, as previously good, positive, healthy relationships become lost in individual uncertainty. Often one partner can blame the other, or feel responsible or guilty about letting the other down, or can swing between these states. People in this position feel that they are in a vacuum and isolated, while the world around appears to be moving on.

As well as treating the physical symptoms, our homeopathic remedies address the mental and emotional processes that our clients are experiencing. The remedies help release pent-up emotions, and this in turn helps people feel released and able to see and feel more clearly – basically to feel a lot better. We often find that couples admit to having lost their sex life and mutual connection, and through our treatment these are re-established.

So, do not simply accept the diagnosis of unexplained infertility – there often is a reason, and there is much that can be done!

7 'THINGS AREN'T QUITE HOW THEY USED TO BE AFTER CONTRACEPTION/FIRST BABY/ TRAUMA/GRIEF …'

Most women expect physical and emotional changes over time, and in many cases these are normal and do not affect overall wellbeing or fertility. Sometimes, however, women are subject to circumstances, medication or trauma that have a negative impact – affecting them physically and emotionally and often standing in the way of them achieving a pregnancy. Women may not link these changes with their difficulty in conceiving or maintaining a pregnancy, but in our experience they can be central to the problem.

The contraceptive pill/hormonal injections/implants

Contraceptives provide control and lifestyle planning, and for most women, once they wish to discontinue them, their cycles quickly re-establish and there is no long-term effect on their fertility. However, there is another group of women for whom the contraceptive hormones do appear to have a long-term effect. These women's cycles do not return to normal and do not properly re-establish. There is a disturbance or change in the cycle.

The disturbance may be obvious, such as periods not returning at all, or being extremely light, perhaps lasting only a day or two whereas they used to be three to four days long. In this instance, it is easy to see the difference, and doctors may be happy to investigate if this is still an issue after six months.

Blood tests may be requested – usually taken on day 21 of the menstrual cycle – and the results will often show that ovulation is unlikely to be occurring or be only just within normal ranges of expected hormonal levels (progesterone in particular) – a borderline acceptable result. An AMH (anti-mullerian hormone) test may also be offered, purportedly to determine the age of the eggs and ovarian reserve. Frequently the AMH test result will be poor and indicate a low ovarian reserve. However, as discussed in detail in Chapter 3, when we see women with this potentially devastating diagnosis, we are able to reassure them that the test result is usually reflective of poor hormone levels rather than absolute egg age.

Almost irrespective of these test results, women are typically given a drug such as clomiphene in an attempt to stimulate ovulation. However when the cycle and its attendant hormones are this quiet and dysfunctional, that may not be sufficient. The next step offered is usually IVF. This is a highly invasive treatment using a range of potent drugs. We find that where the cycle is unbalanced and stuck, these treatments are less likely to be effective – there simply is too little foundation on which to build.

The women we see have typically been through a whole gamut of tests and drug treatments and often IVF, all to no avail. Indeed these measures can even make matters worse. The subsequent cycles often become very irregular, or painful, with accompanying PMT and mood swings. Women may gain weight and feel generally unwell.

More commonly, when coming off the pill or other hormonal contraception, women are relieved to see their cycle returning, and at first may not recognise more subtle changes that have led to it becoming infertile. There may nevertheless be marked differences between how their cycle was before they went on the pill, and how it is since they finished taking it. Perhaps their period used to be a strong five day bleed, and is now a slow-to-medium three day bleed with two light or spotting days. It will usually take a little longer to investigate this type of change, as women in this position won't immediately refer to anyone for help. They see a bleed, assume this means they are ovulating, and keep trying to get pregnant. It is usually only once things have become very stressed or worrying between couples that they decide to look into the problem. Typically we see this happening 18 months to two years after the woman comes off the pill. In this situation, medical tests often do not identify the problem. The test results may appear to be within normal range; however, they still may not be normal for that woman, or may be disproportionate – e.g. one may be at the top end of normal, and another at the lower end – so the hormones don't balance and flow appropriately.

But whether the changes are obvious or more subtle, the infertility diagnosis is often the same: 'unexplained'; low AMH; or just age.

How can contraceptives still be having an effect even after the woman has stopped taking them?

A month after a woman stops taking the contraceptive pill, there is no trace of the drug left in her bloodstream. So what is happening?

The actual process is not clear. There are however things we do know. The pill contains pharmaceutical substances that have been manufactured to mimic human hormones, but actually have a different molecular structure from them. This has to be the case in order for the manufacturers to be able to patent them – it is not legally possible to patent a natural hormone, so the synthetic one has to be sufficiently different so that it can be marketed commercially. However these synthetic hormones have to bind with natural human hormone receptors. These receptors are very sensitive, suitable really just for that individual's own hormones and not for man-made chemicals. In our clients, we have observed that certain pill ingredients appear to have been associated with problems more frequently than others. Synthetic oestrogen is a common ingredient in contraceptive pills, and in hormone replacement therapy, and it seems to have a potent effect on some women's cycles.

Effects are not predictable

The full effects of the combination between synthetic hormones and individual human hormone receptors are not fully known. They certainly appear to vary between women. Not all women react to the pill in the same way; sometimes they are fine for a while before experiencing any adverse symptoms; sometimes such symptoms arise only following another event, such as a pregnancy. This makes predicting the impact on any given individual impossible. However, known side-effects of synthetic oestrogen such as Ethinylestradiol in the contraceptive pill include bloating, fluid retention and depression, and it can increase the risk of breast cancer. This is because in some tissue it can have an effect that may be a thousand times more powerful than natural human oestrogen.

Libido loss can indicate deeper problems

Many women report that taking the pill has lowered their libido. In fact we did see one client who believed that this was how the pill worked – by lowering women's libido so that they don't want intercourse, therefore ensuring they don't get pregnant! There is research that suggests some women may experience this effect long term, even after stopping the pill. This evidence would seem to support the observation we have made from talking to women in our clinic - that ovulatory cycles can be suppressed even after the drugs in the pill are cleared from the bloodstream – a potentially serious finding.

Research suggests that the pill's effect on the libido is due to it causing extra production of a certain protein called sex hormone binding globulin (SHBG). SHBG stores testosterone, and excess production of SHBG therefore causes a reduction in the availability of testosterone – which is important to both male and female libido and reproductive cycles. SHBG also disrupts the production of female pheromones/hormones.

So although we can't be exactly sure what disruption is responsible for the lack of good, strong cycles for some women after they stop taking the pill, there are some clues we have found. We believe the most probable explanation is that it has something to do with the mismatch between the man-made chemical hormones and particularly sensitive human hormone receptors.

CASE STUDY – RUTH

'I had been trying to get pregnant for ten years, and was recommended to see Anne and Claire. I work in a medical environment and really had no faith in homeopathy, but had been nagged by my colleague for so long that I went really so that I could just get a bit of peace and quiet at work – in fact to say, "See, I told you it wouldn't work."

'When Anne and Claire asked me about taking the pill, even the small bit of hope I had that this nonsense treatment might work evaporated – I hadn't taken the pill for over ten years. Yes, my periods were different now, but what did they expect? Doctors laughed at me wanting to get pregnant at my age and said I didn't have a chance, so having any kind of cycle was welcome, and it was bound to be different now, as I was older!

'I dutifully took the homeopathic remedies. My next period didn't come, I took a pregnancy test and couldn't believe it when I saw that it was positive. I now have a lovely little boy. '

Some contraceptives appear to have greater effects than others. We have found that hormonal injections and implants may have more profound effects than the pill. These contraceptives are designed to make a woman sterile for three to six months at a time, and it is commonly known that it in most cases it can take some months after the injections are stopped or the implants removed for the woman's cycles return to normal. In fact the cycles can be very disrupted following use of these contraceptives. Some clients have reported continual bleeds for months before finally having no cycles at all. Others have reported highly irregular cycles. Some have subsequently found it very difficult to conceive.

These forms of contraceptive have been widely used in developing countries to control population growth, and there is a lot of political concern about their long-term effects and the possibility that vulnerable women are at risk of being persuaded into taking them without fully understanding all the side-effects, contraindications and potential impacts.

Again, we cannot say exactly what is happening and why we have seen women whose cycles have never been the same since taking these longer-lasting contraceptives, but we can point to what we have observed and notice that changes appear to happen at a deep hormonal level, and appear to be permanent.

The hormonal coil

The coil is a small device placed in the uterus and designed to prevent a fertilised egg from implanting. Recently-developed examples also incorporate a slow-release hormone called levonorgesterel – a progestogen birth control hormone. Even leaving aside the question of whether or not a woman needs this in addition to the coil's basic function, progestogen has potential negative side-effects that include irregular menstrual cycles, spotting or bleeding between periods, no periods at all, sore breasts, headaches, nausea, dizziness, and bloating or weight gain. As with the pill and other longer-acting contraceptives, we have seen fertility problems persist in some women even after they have had the coil removed.

The good news is that a great deal can be done to help in these cases. Where we think there may be disruption due to the woman reacting to synthetic hormones, we give homeopathic remedies that help to kick-start her correct natural hormonal cycle. This has the effect of resetting the hormonal cascade without the left-over effect from the man-made chemicals. Alongside homeopathic treatment, high quality supplements, especially B vitamins and essential fatty acids, can be important in addressing the issue.

So even if you think you may be in this position, you don't have to just put up with the state of affairs.

Never been the same since first baby – 'I got pregnant first time easily, this time it's been four years and nothing!'

CASE STUDY – CLARE

'When we first decided to have a baby, I got pregnant within three months. The pregnancy was normal, and I loved my little girl. When she was two years old, we thought it would be about the right time to think about having another. But four years later, we were still

trying! At first we thought that maybe we had just been lucky the first time to conceive in only three months – some women do take six to 12 months – but four years! I didn't understand. I hadn't had a single positive pregnancy test. Nothing had changed – we were eating the same, exercising the same. Why on earth was this happening?

'When Anne and Claire said it could be due to hormonal changes that hadn't settled after having my daughter, I didn't really see how that could be true – the pregnancy and birth had been fine. Anyway, I took the homeopathic remedies, and four months later I was pregnant!'

This is another common predicament we see clients facing. As far as they can tell, their lives and lifestyles are no different from when they had their first child, but they can't seem to conceive again. Yes, they are a little busier now that they have a toddler, but they have support from their family and friends – and surely lots of people have two, three or four young children (or more) without a problem?

We find that although many women in this position report feeling okay, even if not back to how they were before, the impact of the first pregnancy and baby is often underestimated. Having a child generally entails a huge transformation for the woman and her family. Physical, hormonal and emotional changes are inevitable, and for some women these do not wholly resolve.

Pregnancy in itself has an enormous effect on a woman's body, with unique changes occurring both before and after the birth. Rebalancing the hormones subsequently can be difficult. There are huge increases during pregnancy in the woman's levels of progesterone and oestradiol (the most potent type of oestrogen), along with increases in growth hormones, cortisol, prostaglandins and relaxin. Physiological changes include increased blood volume, increased cardiac output and increased metabolic rate.

The placenta, which feeds and supports the growing baby, is a major hormone-producing organ in its own right. It is therefore not surprising that after a baby arrives and the placenta is birthed, there are rapid and profound hormonal changes for the woman, with precipitous drops in progesterone and oestrogen.

Other hormones, notably oxytocin and prolactin, are present during birth and increase rapidly after birth to support breastfeeding and bonding between mother and baby.

A combination of events

Our usual finding is that difficulty in conceiving after a previous birth is unlikely to be due to one thing alone – for example it is unlikely to be due just to the woman having initially gone back on the pill after the birth. It is more likely to be down to a combination of a number of different things. These can include not only the woman having initially gone back on the pill, but also stress from looking after a newborn; worry about childcare; exhaustion; and hormones being not quite right following a period of feeling a bit down after the birth.

It is almost a perfect storm of events rather than just one thing. So symptoms and clues may be small, but we specialise in this area, and look carefully for the many factors that may be causing problems. Sometimes there are clearer changes such as intermittent/lighter cycles or depression/low mood, all of which respond very well to homeopathic treatment.

We find depression/low mood has often not been well diagnosed. There is a stigma of shame for women who have had a child and then feel depressed or down. They know that many other women would give their right arm for a baby, and feel they have no right to feel as they do. So they avoid admitting this or seeking help for it, sometimes for many years – not realising that many other mothers feel the same, and similarly don't want to admit it! There can also be an unfair and quite mistaken feeling of failure or guilt.

This is a terrible pity, and when we see women in this position we can usually do a great deal for them. Again, they often say they wish they had known earlier that they could get real help, not just anti-depressants – which, while useful in some circumstances, act to mask symptoms rather than tackle the underlying problems. Typically, in only three to four months of specialist homeopathic treatment, both emotional blocks and physical symptoms shift completely and women can enjoy being a mum again.

We find that once women are well again and the complex hormones rebalanced, they return to having genuinely fertile cycles and can then realistically work toward a new baby.

///

CASE STUDY – LISA

'I had gotten pregnant really easily with my daughter and had a pretty straightforward pregnancy and birth – no problem really. My periods took a long while to come back afterwards and were a bit heavier, but no big deal. We started to try for another baby when my daughter was 18 months old and expected it to happen straightaway, just like before. So when it had been eight months I started to worry.

'My friend had had a baby after seeing Anne and Claire and I thought I had to try something. It wasn't until we went through everything that I realised how lots of aspects of my cycle had gone a bit out since my daughter arrived. I also finally admitted that I was feeling low – I didn't really know why and had just got used to it. It did take some time before I felt really well and back to my old self, and I fell pregnant after six months! I wish I had sorted this out earlier, but I would never let things drift like that again.'

///

Trauma

Everyone experiences a level of trauma in their lives and most people bounce back. Sometimes though the trauma can have more far-reaching effects on the individual. This can arise from a loss/bereavement, from childhood issues, from a difficult pregnancy or birth, or indeed from anything that the individual themselves recognises as having had a significant effect on them. It can be made worse by others minimising the trauma, saying 'everybody had that', or telling them they should 'get over it'.

In our clinic we have seen clients with a range of trauma causes including miscarriage, stillbirth, traumatic birth, childhood abuse, loss of a parent or friend, personal or parental divorce, and so on. A traumatic incident is one that remains with you, where the passage of time hasn't really healed or created a sense of distance and perspective.

CASE STUDY – MARTINE

'Following a terrible shock in my family, my periods stopped completely. I didn't have a period for nearly three years. I accepted this, and didn't really address the issue directly, although I wasn't very happy about it. It seemed like a miracle, then, when I found I was pregnant! I was delighted, and enjoyed every day of my pregnancy, which sailed happily along. Two weeks before my due date, I hadn't felt my baby move for a while, so I went to hospital to be checked. I heard the worst news I could ever hear in my life: my baby's heart had stopped beating.

'The next year was horrible, and made even worse by still having no periods. The doctors had told me that the pregnancy would probably sort out my hormones, but it didn't, and all I could think about was having another baby – but with no periods, how could that ever happen?'

When we saw this woman, it was clear to us that the case was about how shock and trauma – first from her family problems and secondly from the stillbirth of her daughter – had affected her cycle. We gave homeopathic remedies for shock and trauma and her periods returned, regular and strong. She now has a beautiful baby, and is fertile once again.

CASE STUDY – SARAH-ANN

'I had been trying to have a baby for two years. I was young and healthy - I should have been pregnant! When I went for treatment with Anne and Claire, they picked up that I had suffered a loss. My best friend had died seven years earlier in an accident, and it felt like it had happened yesterday. I knew I should get over it but I just couldn't, and I felt overwhelmed every time I thought of it. It was only after I had treatment for the loss and trauma that my cycles changed – I had never realised the effect something that happened so long ago could have on me physically.'

Sadly, too many women experience a traumatic birth, which may lead to postnatal depression, difficulty bonding with their child and a profound fear about any subsequent pregnancy and birth. For some women this can be severe enough to lead to post-traumatic stress disorder (PTSD), symptoms of which may include flashbacks, pervasive anxiety about everyday activities, inability to experience enjoyment – including from sex with their partner – and a sense of isolation and guilt.

It is not simply those births where obviously dramatic problems have occurred that can lead to these problems. Indeed, women can be made to feel that they are 'making a fuss', that 'it wasn't that bad' and that they 'should be happy if they have a live/healthy baby'. This minimisation and failure to recognise the trauma some women have experienced further entrenches and exacerbates the problems experienced by the women and creates a sense of guilt.

///

CASE STUDY – IRENE

'When I saw Anne and Claire I could barely speak about the birth of my son. It had been horrendous. I hadn't even been sure if he was alive when he was born. I had been mismanaged and mistreated during my labour, and I was physically and emotionally a wreck. I had had to pretend that I was okay, though, because everyone said "All that matters is having a healthy baby." But it wasn't all that mattered. Every time I tried to get pregnant after that I miscarried – I was just at my wits' end and wasn't sure if I

could carry on trying.

'Anne and Claire asked me to tell them some of what had happened, but didn't make me relive everything again. I couldn't believe the way that their homeopathic remedies lifted the fear, grief and pure dread. I hadn't really linked the awful birth to me not being able to hold a pregnancy afterwards. Having received treatment, I fell pregnant, and Anne and Claire supported me throughout. My son was born by planned caesarean section, and it was such a positive experience compared with what I had gone through previously.'

We have treated a number of women for this problem - both those who wish to have another child and those who wish simply to feel well again. Trauma, and being 'stuck' as a result, is such a prevalent problem and its causes so diverse that it really deserves a book of its own.

8 EMOTIONS AND STRESS – 'DO THESE REALLY MAKE A DIFFERENCE?'

In treating infertility it is vital to consider the holistic picture of physical and emotional symptoms. Studies have clearly linked stress to fertility problems, so addressing these problems as purely physical ones, as the medical profession so often does, can miss much of the picture and therefore risk missing the cure as well.

CASE STUDY – CATHERINE

'When I was referred by my doctor to the general fertility clinic I felt I was just a series of physical symptoms, a walking uterus! Until I had treatment with Anne and Claire, I had no idea that my grief and feeling of utter hopelessness could actually be helped. They really understood the depth of grief that every month brings. The homeopathic treatment made me feel a lot more balanced, and I began to feel my old, content self again. They also helped my hormonal problems, and now I am pregnant.'

Stress is a term that encapsulates a whole range of emotions. Emotions have the capacity to have a profound effect on every individual, and can cause many symptoms, both physical and mental. Most people, like the one in the case study above, report that when they seek help for infertility, doctors overlook the emotional side of their situation. Couples simply become a series of physical symptoms, and undergo tests that they either 'pass' or 'fail' but feel that they have no control over. Many report feelings similar to those described above, and say, 'I felt they looked at me only as a piece of meat.'

To some extent this is understandable. Medical doctors are simply looking for medical conditions that may explain why the body isn't working as it should be. Their ethos is to prescribe drugs or carry out surgical procedures to correct the problem. If the couple becomes fertile as a result, the problems are over. Couples themselves may also feel that, as a starting point, this is the only way forward. They often view doctors as the people with all the necessary tools to solve their problems.

By the time most couples approach a doctor, emotions between them have already become very strained. Often their relationship is beginning to feel like it has only one purpose – to have a child – and that purpose seems a millions miles away from being achieved. They approach the medical profession confident of their problem being identified and fixed. When the answer isn't readily apparent or makes the situation feel worse – as can happen with a diagnosis of unexplained infertility, drug treatments causing mood swings, or failed IVFs – things can spiral downwards.

It is common for people to suffer doubly; first with their sense of bereavement, and secondly with guilt that they haven't got over their emotions. Couples report the horrible taboo surrounding their inability to have a child.

CASE STUDY – JO

'We were sat in the fertility clinic waiting room, all couples together. No-one looked at anyone else, everyone looked into space, the atmosphere was horrible. A couple of years ago, my mum had cancer, and when I went with her to chemotherapy, people were talking to each other and supportive in the waiting room. This was worse, although I didn't think anything could be.'

CASE STUDY – EVELYN

'I had been trying for seven years to get pregnant, had three rounds of IVF and no positive pregnancy. My friend became pregnant even though she "wasn't really trying". She knew how not having a baby was destroying me. Every time I looked at Facebook there seemed to be another picture of a scan. In the end I couldn't tick the "like" box – I couldn't look without feeling anger and jealousy, and didn't want to feel that. She raged on Facebook about how nasty I was, not celebrating

her success. People joined in, saying that just because I couldn't have a child, that shouldn't stop me being happy for those who could. I am happy for them, but no-one ever thinks I have the right to be sad.'

CASE STUDY – DOROTHY

'I hate Christmas. It's that time for in the in-laws to have a go: "Don't be so selfish. You keep thinking about your holidays and career. Don't deny [my son] the right to have a baby. He's always wanted them, you know." Last year my sister picked up her toddler and said "Come on [toddler] and see Auntie, let's ask her when she is going to get you a little cousin to play with."'

It seems that other people, including family and friends, feel they have a right to comment on and speculate about your plans regarding children, whereas they would recognise this as being completely outrageous if it were about other aspects of your relationship, such as sexual habits! Couples with fertility problems end up covering them up, lying about why they don't have children and pretending they really don't mind having this painful area probed, often in public. It is as if there is a collective sense of shame about not being able to have a child.

A woman will often describe to us her feelings about infertility in terms like these: 'It is the simplest, most basic thing that I am here to do, just have a child, and I can't even do that.' She will also typically feel that she is letting her partner down. They have decided between them that they want children in their relationship; now that she is – as she sees it – letting the man down, were does this leave the relationship? She will often feel that she is letting people down more generally too; not providing playmates for cousins or even friends' children, or grandchildren for grandparents to dote on.

There is often a sense of couples wanting to leave a legacy, a part of themselves intellectually and biologically, as well as handing down family values. They may also want to experience that part of themselves that is a parent. The thought of this not being possible can a lead to a rising sense of panic that they may never achieve their dreams.

Stress and emotions change things on a physical level

Couples clearly feel a great deal of stress when struggling with infertility; but apart from being unpleasant, does the stress really matter?

Stress leads to a state of anxiety, fear or even panic. The natural reaction to these emotions is for the body to attempt to create a state of balance – also referred to as homeostasis. Having such a reaction is not inherently bad; it is normal and useful in the right circumstances. In ancient times, stress would often arise from a dangerous situation such as facing a wild animal about to attack. This would cause the body to set off a series of hormonal signals provoking a 'fight or flight' response;

if you did nothing, you would be in danger, but by either fighting the danger or fleeing from it, you might survive.

This underlying response to stress still exists. The hypothalamus is the part of the brain responsible for producing chemicals to control the stress response. On receiving a signal that there is a stressor, it produces corticotropin-releasing hormone (CRH), which stimulates the anterior pituitary gland to release adrenocorticotropic hormone into the bloodstream. This in turn binds to the adrenal gland to release cortisol. Cortisol has a widespread impact on the body. It redistributes glucose (sugar energy) into critical areas such as the brain and the heart, and away from areas it considers non-critical for survival such as digestive system and reproductive organs.

Once the danger has passed, and the body no longer feels stress, its natural feedback system switches these responses off. If the stress was a physical one (such as running away from the wild animal), the body will have used up the extra chemicals (by running or fighting). However, if the stress resulted in no physical activity, the chemicals still have to be cleared by the body, so for a while longer, even after the stress has passed, the body has extra work to do in eliminating this toxic load before fully returning to normal. Once returned to normal, the body is able to give energy to digestion and reproduction, or other secondary activities other than direct survival. This is why many people feel better after visiting a gym or going running, or any physical activity to relieve stress.

When the stress is constant – and in this instance we are looking specifically at anxiety and fear about infertility – it is apparent how these mechanisms are at work all the time. This is occurring even when couples try to put their problem out of their minds. It may be to one side while they have a holiday or a lovely evening with friends, but deep-seated concern or worry will still be causing a stress response, even if perhaps to a lesser degree.

One way of testing how stressed you are about a situation is to think how it would feel if that worry wasn't there. If you feel a surge of lightness and peace , then that is how much stress you are carrying about a situation. We often get so used to our worries that we don't always realise how they are influencing us, and we are therefore used to the chemical stress response of not feeling light and at peace.

Research on stress and fertility

In 2009, researchers at the University of California, Berkeley found more evidence supporting the idea that stress can cause sexual dysfunction and infertility.[11]

Until that point, it was known that there was some effect from the stress 'fight or flight' response creating the hormonal cascade outlined above, which includes the release of cortisol. Cortisol inhibits gonadotropin-releasing hormone (GnRH), which is the body's main sex hormone. Suppressing this influences ovulation, sperm count and libido. GnRH is produced in the hypothalamus, and it then goes on to stimulate the pituitary gland to produce luteinising hormone (LH) and follicle-stimulating hormone (FSH). These in turn stimulate the production of testosterone and estradiol – the hormones that lead to sperm production in men and egg production in women.

---

[11] University of California, Berkeley (2009) 'Stress Puts Double Whammy on Reproductive System.' Fertility Science Daily. 29 June 2009.

What the scientists at Berkeley discovered is that there is an additional mechanism at work. Stress increases the levels in the brain of a reproductive hormone called gonadotropin inhibitory hormone (GnIH). This has a direct inhibitory effect on the critical GnRH, in effect stopping the reproductive hormones in their tracks.

So, in short, stress causes interference in three key ways:

- releasing cortisol, which inhibits GnRH;

- prioritising essential bodily functions over reproduction; and

- producing GnIH, which inhibits key reproductive hormones.

It is therefore vital to address stress and negative emotions. It is not sufficient to think of infertility as a physical problem alone.

What can homeopathy do for you?

The stress feedback cycle is a loop. Stress creates the cascade of hormones, leading to cortisol and GnIH being released; these cause the body to prioritise a 'fight or flight' mechanism, using these hormones by energising muscle, often at the cost of other routine bodily functions; the body then loops around to re-check the status of the stress. Is the stress gone? If yes, then it calms back down to normal. If the stress is still there, then it begins the loop again.

If the source of stress is a single attack, it is easy to see how the effects will pass. However, in today's busy and demanding world, we are constantly living with stress that the body will pick up – unemployment, difficulties at work, money worries, housing problems, health issues, bereavement, social pressures etc. So relaxing, and having a balanced mind and body, is difficult.

The particular stresses around fertility can be almost uniquely overwhelming. Couples often feel a complex array of emotions: the lack of control over the outcome, the personal feelings of failure, the grief of loss every monthly cycle, the fear that they may never achieve their goal, etc. Alongside this, couples also experience immense social and family pressures and can often feel outcast and isolated. So the stress cascade of damaging hormones in infertility cases can run almost constantly, as there is no natural 'out', no natural stopping or resolution of these feelings.

Homeopathy can help in these situations where there is no natural break by dissipating the hormones quickly before they become part of a larger loop. This means that not only do couples feel more balanced, the body actually stops the unwanted hormone cascade. By intervening and creating balance – homeostasis – in this way, homeopathy can actually help the body to have less of a physical reaction to the stress. It is then much more able to dedicate resources to creating more balanced and effective fertility hormones. The ongoing effect of this is that you feel much better and much more in control.

Unlike conventional drug therapy, homeopathic remedies are able to be used intelligently by the body. Remedies are prescribed by the practitioner when they feel a person is out of balance. There is no single 'stress' remedy like an anti-depressant; instead we analyse the prevalent emotions and how the particular individual reacts to stress. Commonly we see anger, resentment, jealously, anxiety, inadequacy, feelings of failure – we have a wealth of different remedies for different aspects of each of these emotional responses.

Giving the correct remedy not only helps the person recover from the situation and feel better much quicker, it also has a long-term benefit. Clients report feeling much better not just in that moment, but all the time. This is because the remedy is working with the body's natural ability to balance. It enables the body to find that balance and switch off the stress loop much more quickly.

〰〰〰

CASE STUDY – FIONA

'My first IVF worked perfectly, and two years later we decided to have another child. When six further rounds of IVF failed, I was beginning to feel like this would never happen. I was diagnosed with unexplained infertility, which felt awful. If they didn't know the cause, how could anything be fixed? If I hadn't already had my first child, I might have felt suicidal. It was now 14 years in all we had been struggling with this. IVF didn't seem to be working now, and all I could think was how many years of my life I had wasted. Instead of enjoying my daughter, I was constantly unhappy, going into or coming out of unsuccessful IVF. I was moody and on anti-depressants and sleeping pills. The more I wasn't enjoying life, the more it was making me depressed and guilty that I was wasting what I had, but I couldn't seem to do anything about it. My husband I were together still, but to be

honest we just couldn't be bothered having sex anymore – it was only for fertility, and that was always a failure, so what was the point?

    'It was out of desperation that I went to Claire and Anne. I really didn't know what else to do. I had been recommended to see them, and to me it was a shot to nothing. When they talked about stress and emotions, I wasn't very interested. It all sounded a bit woolly, like they were avoiding the issue of my unexplained infertility. I just wanted to be pregnant.

    'I took my remedies, and was surprised when my periods changed. I realised that my cycle hadn't been right after all. But the most unexpected side-effect was that I felt much better. In fact, so much better that my doctor was happy to help me to come off my anti-depressants. I was able to enjoy my little girl, and felt much more at ease with whether or not I had another baby. Although I knew I still would love one, somehow it didn't feel as desperate. My husband and I even found we were having sex for fun from time to time! I felt more in control and much better about the future, whether or not I could become pregnant naturally. Even when considering further IVF, I felt more in control, and not so panicky.'

Conventional stress-reducing drugs – anti-depressants – simply switch off and dull particular parts of a feedback system, which has a blanket effect – often described as 'just feeling nothing'.

They don't aim to solve the root of the problem, they just hold people in a place until the problem either disappears or is resolved through another method. Although they definitely have their place and uses, they can be quite a blunt instrument, and are not always a good precursor for pregnancy.

Stress, the immune system, fertility and holistic therapy

When treating people, we find it is important to take a holistic view. Those coming to see us for fertility or hormonal issues often describe other apparently unrelated symptoms or problems. All such symptoms can be useful clues, so it is often necessary to ask a client about their general health, childhood and family health history. These things give further indications about general susceptibility or weaknesses in the body – such as a weak chest, digestive disorders such as IBS, or eczema – which from time to time will cause them repeated problems in their life. These recurrent issues may flare up in times of stress, on holiday or at certain times of year such as winter or Christmas.

The link between stress and the immune system has been widely studied, and it is generally accepted that when stress is detected, a physical biochemical response occurs that impacts on the immune system. This leaves people more susceptible to pick up general infections and viruses that are around at the time. Often people will also experience ill health in the same area of the body each time – their 'weak' spot.

CASE STUDY – CAROLINE

'My husband and I feel like we have been struggling with infertility, everyone around us getting pregnant and failed IVF forever. Last winter things reached a crisis when he was talking about ending our marriage. All I could think was that he was going off with a younger woman to have a family. I felt destroyed. I couldn't cope. I had always suffered with viral infections during the winter and last year was the worst, resulting in hospitalisation and many months of antibiotic treatment. I have now been prescribed constant antibiotics in case I get ill again. I really don't feel I need them, as I feel much better in myself now that I have dealt with the underlying stress, but the doctors don't see how the shock of last year could have affected me.'

In the standard medical worldview, each body system is considered and treated separately. This is particularly apparent when a GP refers a patient to various specialists, each of whom concentrates on his or her own particular area of expertise. The in-depth knowledge that these specialists can bring may be invaluable, but it is not always easy to link from one specialist area to another. So, while this can be an appropriate approach, it definitely has its limitations.

Doctors are used to dealing with multiple health problems piecemeal, and directing patients to a different person to investigate each puzzle piece. This can be exhausting and repetitive for the patient, and risks losing sight of the importance of underlying emotional causes for physical symptoms, or emotional trauma arising from physical events. These problems are not easy to address or fix, and if they are not within the area of the particular specialist seen, may be put to one side.

This is why holistic therapy is so important. Homeopathy works by getting the body to rebalance on all levels. Although we often see clients who initially feel that they have clear issues in one specific area of their life – wanting to be pregnant – usually the lines quickly become blurred. The physical problems attached to fertility cause emotional problems, then those emotional problems – e.g. from a relationship with attendant deep sense of failure – affect the physical weak points, including fertility, creating a vicious circle.

CASE STUDY – VICKY

'I had always had a bad chest. Even as a young girl, I used to have chest infections and would be off school with horrible coughs. These had become worse in the last couple of years, and I had been referred to various specialists until reaching a top professor at the chest hospital.

'The symptoms were changing a bit as well. I would go to pick up my little girl from school feeling fine, then suddenly out of nowhere I would collapse in the playground, unable to catch my breath. I would have to go to hospital in an ambulance, then over the next two to three days I would gradually feel better and could come home. These episodes were getting more common too.

'I had always suffered badly with endometriosis too. I had originally been told that I would never get pregnant, but with the help of my fertility specialist I did everything I could to get the symptoms reduced, and in the end I did have three lovely children. However, recently the endometriosis had got also much worse. Although I kept telling each of the specialists about the other problem with my chest, they seemed completely uninterested.

'After one horrible episode of being unable to breathe, a doctor who was visiting from another country examined my chest and asked if I had any history of endometriosis. When I told him I had, he carried out some other tests. It turned out that the endometriosis had wrapped itself around my lungs. On each period, the endometriosis tightened around my lungs and caused the problem with my breathing. It wasn't two problems, it was one! As soon as this became clear, I was given a different treatment, and I have been fine for over a year now.'

Although some people with fertility issues undertake counselling or obtain other forms of emotional support, this is not always the case, and it may not form part of the treatment of the physical problems looked at elsewhere. The help is still piecemeal. It is also more commonly undertaken where the emotional issues have become unavoidable or are considered 'acceptable' – such as overcoming childhood abuse or family issues. Where the deep emotional pain comes 'just' from not having a child, many people outside of this situation see it as something to 'get over' and not be 'so self-indulgent' about. So seeking help for such a problem can feel like admitting weakness. Feelings of selfishness and/or weakness can make people in this position feel more worthless. They can experience feelings of failure, not just on a physical level for being apparently unable to have a family, but also on an emotional level for being unable to cope with this.

By treating from a holistic perspective, observing which aspect is most prominent and giving homeopathic remedies to allow the body to break out of this debilitating loop, we can bring about a total rebalance. Instead of spinning quicker and tighter trying to find peace, the body is able to balance the stress hormones naturally. The person feels back in control – without effort.

Another aspect of homeopathy that is unique is that when addressing mental and emotional problems, we need only to understand the 'stuck' areas. This is what good counselling will also do – but then it will go on to probe and talk around those areas, which can take a long time and can be too painful for some people, who may feel it is just revisiting and raking up the negative emotions, as it often involves going over issues that can seem intractable.

As homeopaths, by contrast, we ask only the questions we need to ask in order for us to understand what the emotions feel like, what they are related to and exactly how they affect the client. We then give a remedy that clears and gives a good perspective on that 'stuck' or conflicted area. Homeopathic treatment is quicker and less painful than counselling. It doesn't avoid the issues, but instead taps into the natural ability of the mind and body to heal themselves.

Nearly all of our clients come to us seeking treatment for physical fertility issues – which may include the unhelpful diagnosis of 'unexplained infertility'. They know they have mental and emotional pain, but expect these to be the silent, personal hell that they as a couple must endure. Almost all of them are amazed that we ask about and offer to help with the mental and emotional issues as well as the physical ones – and even more amazed that following our treatment these seemingly intractable problems feel so much more under control and improved.

CASE STUDY – KAYE

'Although my IVF was successful, I had the misfortune of a stillbirth. The grief and pain were beyond belief, and I could hardly speak. I had to consider further IVF almost straightaway, so I went to see Claire and Anne to get help for my body to recover quickly from the trauma, so that I could start the procedures again. I didn't want to speak

about the pain, it was beyond awful – nothing could take that away. I wanted to concentrate on physical recovery and further IVF.

'What surprised me was that I could speak a little about my feelings, and it seemed they understood. I was very reluctant to take any remedies. How could little white tablets help this enormous pain? It felt at first as if it was minimising the trauma. But after I did take the remedies, I found that I could cry and feel a little better, not just cry and cry. I could find short intervals in the day that felt bright. Although the pain was there, it was less palpable. I was able to begin to grieve, and also to begin to look forward with balance.

'Along with counselling and support from doctors, the homeopathy was amazing.'

Even when major emotional events occur, such as that described above, the mind and body look to find balance, and they do this through a natural process of grieving. When shock and trauma have been extreme or prolonged, time alone can't heal them. They need to be dissipated through treatment; then the mind, body and spirit are able to start to recover.

There are other useful ways to help manage emotional issues, and we often suggest to clients the following:

- Meditation. There are many different types of mediation, and it is a matter of finding out which one suits each individual. Mindfulness meditation has been shown to be highly beneficial for a lot of people, and there are many affordable CDs available to help practise this.

• Yoga. Meditative yoga practices can also be very helpful in releasing stress and emotions and developing positive breathing and relaxation techniques.

• Dietary changes. Another approach that can help is reducing intake of sugar and white carbohydrates that can lead to sugar spikes and cravings and affect mood. There are a number of natural supplements available that can help to support depleted body systems – these may need to target the immune system, the digestion, the thyroid etc.

So many people suffer needlessly for a long time, thinking there is nothing they can do. With homeopathy, the part of the mental and emotional state that is stuck can be helped to become clear and free. Again people tell us, 'I wish I'd known earlier' – and understandably so. It's not great to suffer when there is a process of healing available.

9 IVF – 'CAN ANYTHING IMPROVE MY CHANCES OF IVF WORKING?'

Broadly speaking, IVF has a success rate of live births of about 25%. However, there are certainly things that can be done to improve the chances of it working.

IVF is aimed at solving the initial problem of conception, and at this it is often successful. However the subsequent growth and development is something for which the body's own hormones are needed. IVF uses synthetic hormones and drugs to stimulate the eggs; these are then extracted from the body, combined with sperm outside the body, then transferred back into the uterus. Further basic synthetic hormones (e.g. progestogen) are given to increase the progesterone levels, with the aim of helping the pregnancy hold, then the body's response is awaited.

In our clinic we have seen many couples who have had repeated IVF cycles that have failed, often for unknown reasons, even when the embryos were considered to be of top quality. In truth, IVF looks only at putting the egg and the sperm together; there are many other things it does not address that are needed to ensure a successful term pregnancy.

Hormonal changes are continual from the initial conception. These are to allow implantation of the egg, sufficient blood supply, formation of the placenta (placentation), development of the foetus, including the internal organs (organogenesis), and so on. Levels of hormones such as progesterone, oestrogen and HCG (human chorionic gonadotropin – the hormone detected by pregnancy tests – have to rise and balance in order for pregnancy to continue. The conditions for this to occur are established when the eggs are still in their initial development phase, two to three months prior to the IVF taking place. Although the IVF drugs stimulate the ovaries to produce a number of eggs, what happens both before and after that is incredibly important.

For our clients who have decided to try IVF, preparation three to four months in advance seems to have given a substantially better chance of success. With our homeopathic remedies, we aim to create a balanced hormonal cycle, which may include ovulation, strong endometrium (womb lining) and good peaks and troughs of oestrogen and progesterone levels. This helps establish the best basis for the body to respond to the fertilised egg after it is returned to the uterus to implant and begin the necessary series of changes.

CASE STUDY – LENA

'When we did our first IVF attempt, I thought that the drugs would sort out my cycle – the clinic said they would take over my cycle and do all the work of getting eggs ready and fertilised. I hadn't realised how important it was to get my period regular so that the IVF had something to work off. It took nearly six months to get my cycle ready.'

Does it make any difference where I have IVF? Aren't all the clinics the same?

The choice of IVF clinic can make a huge difference. There is a great range of options available. There are, for instance, some clinics that specialise in working with your natural cycle, offering to minimise the drugs used. They collect the one or two eggs naturally produced during a cycle and then, after fertilisation and transfer back into the uterus, allow your body to do the rest naturally. At the other extreme, some clinics offer to take over your body's cycle completely, first shutting down your normal hormonal system using the contraceptive pill, then stimulating it again with a range of other drugs – which can have emotional side-effects and run the risk of hyper-stimulation. Drugs such as blood-thinners, steroids and synthetic hormones are commonly used.

Each individual has a different response to the drugs, and while some IVF clinics monitor their clients closely and adjust the regime accordingly, others tend to have a more generic approach. It is important that you pick the right clinic, clinician and approach to suit you. Many of our clients who have undertaken IVF have told us that they have felt 'pressurised through fear' into having as many drugs and as much intervention as their clinic offered, when this may not have been the most appropriate route for them.

Those who are more sensitive to hormone and drug treatment are particularly suited to those regimes that minimise their use. These seem to allow their body's natural hormones to wake, function and work more successfully.

CASE STUDY – MARY

'We had our first three cycles of IVF at a clinic that pretty much threw every drug possible at me. To be honest, I thought that if I had everything possible, I would have the best chance. But although I produced lots of eggs that looked good, nothing took. We were devastated. Then my cycle just went haywire – I didn't ovulate regularly or even get my period when I expected. I felt like a mess, and I was so volatile emotionally. Anne and Claire got my cycle not just back on an even keel but even better than it had been before – and I stopped biting my husband's head off! I decided to go to a different IVF clinic, and this time picked one that used fewer drugs and tailored it more to me. Anne and Claire gave extra remedies for each aspect of the IVF cycle, and finally, success! Can't tell you how thrilled we are!'

We are extremely experienced and careful in giving homeopathic remedies that support the individual IVF cycle, tailored to the particular woman and her history and the type of IVF cycle chosen. We avoid giving remedies that could balance hormones and potentially reduce the effectiveness of any drugs given in the IVF cycle. Instead we give specially-selected supportive remedies that aim to enhance particular functions such as building endometrium, enabling implantation, and initial embryo development.

Understanding IVF

As mentioned, IVF consists essentially of extracting eggs from the woman, combining these with sperm, and returning a fertilised egg or eggs (embyro) to the uterus to await events. However, before IVF is considered, clinicians may suggest drugs such as clomiphene or tamoxifen to stimulate ovulation. These drugs work by blocking oestrogen receptors, so that the body is tricked into thinking it has too little oestrogen and reacts by producing more. They are very commonly given even in cases where it is known from hormone tests and scans that ovulation is already occurring. They are a comparatively cheap, low-intervention first step, and we know from our clients that this can feel like a one-size-fits-all approach that ignores their personal circumstances. A typical comment is, 'I have no idea why they gave me clomiphene. I know I am ovulating, and so do they. That isn't the problem!'

As with all drugs, side-effects are possible. Some of these may be transitory and relatively minor – such as bloating, headaches and mild nausea. Others may be more serious – such as extreme mood changes, hot flushes/sweating and ovarian hyper-stimulation syndrome (OHSS), a potentially life-threatening condition discussed in more detail below. A downright unhelpful side-effect seen in some women is an increase in the thickness of vaginal mucus – which can make it very difficult for sperm to pass into the uterus, making fertilisation and pregnancy highly unlikely!

How women respond to these first-line drug therapies is very individual. Some experience few problems and respond readily, increasing their ovulatory hormones and producing receptive, fertile eggs. Typically we find this is in cases where the hormones are close to being in the correct balance. Other women, particularly those who are either highly sensitive to drugs or whose own hormones are more markedly unbalanced, do not find these drugs helpful, and in our experience they can increase the dysfunction within the woman's cycle.

Once women have tried these drugs and been unsuccessful, they may be offered IVF. This is most commonly used where there is 'unexplained infertility' or damage to the fallopian tubes (the tubes through which the eggs must travel from the ovary in order to reach the uterus). There are two main protocols – the long protocol and the short protocol.

In the long protocol, the clinician takes over the cycle completely. Many clinicians prefer this, as they feel it may be more successful. Two approaches are common – one where the woman is given the contraceptive pill for a month followed by a drug described as a down regulator to suppress her ovaries; the other where the stage of giving the pill is skipped and the woman begins treatment immediately with the down regulator. Some clinics no longer take the first of these approaches, as it can be too effective at suppressing the natural hormones and reduce the woman's capacity to respond to the subsequent drugs and produce high-quality eggs. In our clients we have observed that the use of the contraceptive pill in the long protocol seems to be detrimental to successful IVF. Once it is determined that the down regulator – the drug to suppress the ovaries – has worked, the woman is then given a further range of hormones to stimulate egg production until scans determine that sufficient eggs have been produced. The number of eggs produced will vary enormously from woman to woman and depending on how many drugs have been given.

In the short protocol, the woman moves directly onto the stimulating drugs. The short protocol is therefore faster, involves taking fewer drugs and works a little more alongside the natural cycle.

While clinics may be pleased to see a large number of eggs being produced, this may be likened to hothousing or forced growing; and while some women respond well, it is clear from our experience that this focus on number of eggs does not necessarily lead to eggs capable of creating a successful pregnancy. Perhaps this ought to be viewed less as a numbers game. It seems logical that the two to three eggs closest to ovulation at the start of treatment are likely to be the most capable of developing into embryos and onwards. To use drug therapy to drag out excessive numbers of immature eggs appears unnecessary and counterproductive. It also underplays the enormous emotional cost to the couple. The drugs given and the stresses involved lead to a real rollercoaster of emotions and can place great strain on a couple's relationship. A typical comment we have heard from a male partner is, 'She just gets crazy! I can't talk to her – she just seems to hate me. I don't know how much more of this we can go through.'

Some clinics have developed what is often termed 'natural' IVF. This avoids or minimises use of most of the drugs commonly associated with IVF and instead simply monitors the woman's cycle, harvests the one or two eggs that are naturally produced, and works mainly with the normal hormonal cycle. This can be a very valuable approach – especially for those who are sensitive to drugs and artificial hormones – but the woman's cycle must be regular and strong in order for it to be a realistic possibility.

We have worked with clients where we have established a strong, balanced cycle but other problems have remained, such as scarring of the fallopian tubes or male sexual performance problems. In these cases, natural IVF is then a positive and helpful option that overcomes what might otherwise be insurmountable obstacles.

As discussed in Chapter 5, where sperm quality or volume is a problem, there is a variant on IVF called intra-cytoplasmic sperm injection (ICSI) that may be offered. This involves the clinician selecting an apparently healthy sperm and injecting it directly into the egg. This procedure does not improve the underlying quality or volume of sperm and we would recommend taking steps to address those issues first, so that ideally a natural conception takes place, or at least so that more options are available.

For lesbian couples, intra-uterine insemination (IUI) can be offered. This enables the sperm to be inserted directly into the uterus through a small tube placed into the vagina and through the cervix. Some lesbian couples may be offered additional aspects of typical IVF, such as drugs to stimulate ovulation, however these carry risks of side-effects and may not be needed where a normal ovulatory cycle exists.

Ovarian Hyperstimulation Syndrome (OHSS)

The most serious side-effect of IVF is OHSS. This occurs where the body reacts too strongly to the stimulating drugs, and usually begins around four to five days after eggs have been harvested. It is a potentially life-threatening complication caused by the IVF drugs, although most cases are mild or moderate. It is, however, relatively common to experience some degree of OHSS; in fact around one third of all IVF cycles cause mild OHSS. In these cases the stimulating medication has to be stopped and the planned cycle abandoned (although the embryo may be frozen for use in a future cycle).

As many as 2% of IVF cycles lead to severe OHSS. This serious inflammatory condition requires urgent medical care. Symptoms include rapid weight gain, bloating, fluid retention, scanty/dark urine, abdominal pain and nausea and vomiting. If very severe, the condition can lead to thromboembolism, renal damage, shortness of breath/respiratory distress and ovarian torsion/twisting.

Clinics providing IVF have a responsibility to monitor their patients' wellbeing and reaction to the powerful medications used, and should offer care, advice and support to anyone experiencing any of the OHSS symptoms. It is of course better to avoid such serious complications and to consider what level of medication each couple is willing to take, should they undergo IVF treatment.

10 EARLY MISCARRIAGE/REPEATED MISCARRIAGE – 'IS THIS EVER GOING TO WORK?'

Most women have had at least one miscarriage. It can be a normal part of natural selection and development – not all eggs are viable and not all pregnancies are destined to continue. However, this is not to minimise the emotional devastation that can be caused, particularly for those couples who experience repeated miscarriage. Far too many well-meaning friends and family members, and even some doctors, are prone to say that a miscarriage may have been for the best, and that there was probably something wrong with the baby anyway. This is often without any factual basis, and can just compound the hurt.

Currently in the UK, those couples who experience three or more miscarriages may ask their doctor for referral for an investigation as to why this may have happened. In the vast majority of cases, no apparent cause is found. When couples are looking for answers, it can be frustrating to have this happen – although, on the positive side, it can reassure them that there are no inherited chromosomal abnormalities. But having no immediate and obvious solution can be hard.

Hormone imbalance

One of the most important factors in miscarriage that we see in our clinic is hormonal imbalance. Once a woman has actually conceived, a whole series of hormonal changes occur in her body every single day. HCG (human chorionic gonadotropin) surges, as does progesterone. Oestrogen increases and relaxin and prolactin are produced. Cortisol and growth hormones are increased to enable the foetus to develop. All these, and other, hormones are needed for a successful pregnancy, but it is not enough for them to be present – they must be present at appropriate and proportionate levels and they must adjust and change continually.

If a women enters pregnancy without having a good, strong hormonal cycle, her ability to respond to these day-to-day changes can be diminished. In our clinic, where we naturally encounter a disproportionate number of people with problems, we see many women with a history of disrupted hormonal cycles who are seemingly unable to carry a pregnancy.

Ensuring a good, balanced cycle before pregnancy can help, and we give remedies to try to get the body to respond correctly to heightened hormonal responses. We also examine a whole range of other potential issues, some of which are described below.

Insufficient blood supply?

One test that can be carried out is to measure the blood supply that will be available to the baby. When an egg is fertilised, it travels down the fallopian tube to the uterus and then attempts to burrow itself into the uterine lining. This is a very delicate process where the embryo has to line up exactly with the spot into which it aims to implant. It then burrows in – sometimes releasing a small amount of blood from the lining – and attempts to create connections and remodel the endometrial lining to connect to the mother's blood supply and eventually form the placenta. Obviously at these early stages things are on a microscopically small scale, and the blood has to squeeze through tiny, delicate tubes. If the blood is essentially too thick to perform this process efficiently, then the embryo cannot grow appropriately and continue, resulting in a miscarriage.

In the relatively small proportion of cases where a reason for miscarriage is found in medical tests, this is the most common one – that the women's blood supply is impaired or the blood is too thick. The recommended treatment is often to take a mini aspirin (75 mg) daily with food, which has the effect of slightly thinning the blood. There is some very limited evidence that this may slightly reduce the risk of miscarriage in cases where blood supply is known to be a problem – but it is not of general use for women who have had recurrent miscarriage for other reasons. Some women may have heard or read about treatment with other drugs that are clinically used as blood thinners, such as Clexane or Enoxaparin. However, we know of no evidence that these stronger drugs actually offer any additional help in preventing miscarriage.

Antiphospholipid syndrome

Antiphospholipid syndrome (APS) is an autoimmune condition thought to be responsible for approximately one in six cases of recurrent miscarriage. Phospholipids are a key component of the cells of the body, and if the body begins to produce antibodies to them, this leads to increased clotting (coagulation) of the blood, which can impede the development of any growing embryo. It is not known what causes APS. Treatment usually involves taking blood-thinning agents such as aspirin and heparin. Additionally we recommend homeopathic remedies to improve blood flow.

Super-fertility?

A recent small-scale study from the Netherlands pointed to a new potential cause of recurrent miscarriage – super-fertility.[12] The researchers examined the lining of the womb in women who were known to have had recurrent miscarriage and found that it responded equally to low-quality embryonic tissue as to high-quality embryonic tissue. This was despite the fact that such low-quality tissue would have little or no chance of developing. This contrasts with the results from women known to have had successful pregnancies. Their womb lining responded positively only to high-quality embryonic tissue. The conclusion of the study was that some women are super-fertile – their bodies fail to discriminate between 'high-quality' embryos and 'low-quality' embryos.

Although this was a small-scale study, we ourselves have seen a small number of clients for whom this appears to be the issue. These women typically present as getting pregnant every time they have unprotected sex at a fertile point in their cycle. There should be a natural variation in the production of eggs and sperm – this enables nature to 'try out' different combinations. The natural course of events is for the body to reject immediately any combination of egg and sperm that won't actually work. However, these women seem to hang

---

[12] *Weimar et al 2012.*

on to such imperfect combinations for several weeks, even though they cannot progress to a full pregnancy. This can be heart-breaking. We work by giving constitutional homeopathic remedies to try to get the woman's body to become more balanced. This will enable the womb lining to respond appropriately and naturally to each embryo.

Development barriers?

It can be important to note when miscarriages occur, to see if they continually coincide with the same stage of gestational development. For example, if they always occur at five to six weeks, the suggests that the reason relates to the formation of the heart. This is actually quite a common time for miscarriages to occur, as this is a particularly complicated part of the foetus's development! In this instance, we may give particular remedies to support this stage of development.

Combination of factors?

Many other causes of recurrent miscarriage have been proposed, and for some couples a combination of factors may well be involved. Certainly hormonal imbalance, including PCOS, can be an issue, as can chromosomal abnormalities. Such abnormalities are thought to be implicated in up to half of miscarriages, although couples may be reassured that they are usually a one-off problem rather than an ongoing one.

It has been suggested that natural killer cells also play a role in recurrent miscarriage, but the evidence for this is very thin and highly controversial. The most comprehensive recent review found that there was no value in testing for natural killer cells/immune factors and that the suggested treatment options (such as immunisation with paternal leukocytes and treatment with intravenous immune globulin (IVIG)) do not in fact help in cases of unexplained recurrent miscarriage. In our experience such treatment is expensive, traumatic and ineffective.

///

CASE STUDY – JO AND ANDY

'We had had four miscarriages. There wasn't a pattern to it – one at six weeks, one at eight weeks, one at ten weeks and one at five weeks. We were just desperate to have a baby, but we were also frightened – we just couldn't face the prospect of becoming pregnant again and then going through yet another terrible loss. We were both stressed out to the max, and Jo's cycle had gone all over the place – we thought it Jo's PCOS coming back. Anne and Claire recognised right away that there were a lot of things that had to be addressed – some of which we hadn't even considered. They tackled our stress levels – which were much higher than we had even realised – and got started on getting Jo's cycle back into shape. It was such a relief to talk to people who dealt with the emotional and physical side of things together. It was some eight months before we fell pregnant again, and each week felt fraught with difficulty. At our early pregnancy scan at eight weeks, the pregnancy was viable and growth was right

for the gestation. We continued homeopathic treatment throughout the pregnancy, and our incredible, beautiful baby girl was born.'

\\\

Emotional issues

Recurrent miscarriage is one of the most traumatising experiences any couple can face. The toxic mix of hope, anxiety, fear and grief is awful; and friends and relatives quickly run out of anything comforting or supportive to say. What's more, couples often receive disparate and confusing advice after miscarriage, with many being told to wait at least six months before trying for another pregnancy – although in fact this is not backed up by any research, and couples can really begin trying again whenever they feel ready.

We find that, unless blood supply/clotting has been shown to be the problem, the medical profession has few answers to offer. Many couples are advised to take the mini aspirin alongside food, simply because it is one of the few treatments that has been shown to work in some cases, and has relatively few complications. But often this is ineffective and provides no solution.

In our clinic we provide a space for counselling and support of the grief, and give good homeopathic remedies to help dissipate the negative emotions and stress hormones, as well as helping with the physical issues. Our approach is, as always, to get the body to rebalance itself correctly. By getting the original and correct feedback system working, we have a high success rate and turn around many couples who felt they had no chance of holding a successful pregnancy.

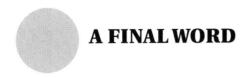

A FINAL WORD

It is worth reiterating that generally in our homeopathy fertility clinic we see people who have come to us feeling that they have no other option left. Often they have been written off by a general fertility clinic as being too old to have a baby (age 40 to 45), or conventional medical treatment just won't seem to work for them. Many of them have been told that their problems are intractable. We give no promises; we are always honest and open in our consultations; and together with our clients we discuss and agree treatment plans and expectations and keep a close track of how things progress.

We see people with a wide range of problems. Most of our clients do not come with straightforward issues. Some are actively seeking to become pregnant, others wish to maximise their chances of pregnancy in the future, e.g. by having PCOS treated. Many are largely in the dark about the issues involved, having previously been given little information about hormonal cycles, fertility or what their choices are.

The fact that we often see successful outcomes in these disproportionately complex and problematic cases, where doctors have typically offered little hope, is what has given us the push to write this book. We would urge anyone who finds themselves in the position of suffering seemingly intractable fertility problems not simply to accept that 'nothing can be done'. There may be nothing that your current clinician can do, but others may be able to help. Even at an early stage, when you have not long been trying to get pregnant, you might find it worthwhile to try homeopathy – before you consider embarking on more expensive medical treatment, and before stress and worry really set in.

You never know, it might just change everything!

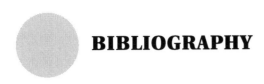

BIBLIOGRAPHY

Alper M, Smith L, Sills E (2009) 'Ovarian Hyperstimulation Syndrome: Current Views On Pathophysiology And Risk.' *Journal of Experimental and Clinical Assisted Reproduction.* Volume 10 p.6:3.

Agarwal A, Makker K and Sharma R (2008) 'Clinical Relevance Of Oxidative Stress In Male Factor Infertility: An Update.' *American Journal of Reproductive Immunology.* 59(1):2-11.

Clark P, Walker I, Langhorne P, Crichton L, Thomson A, Greaves M, et al. (2010) 'SPIN (Scottish Pregnancy Intervention) Study: A Multicentre, Randomised Controlled Trial Of Low-Molecular-Weight Heparin And Low-Dose Aspirin In Women With Recurrent Miscarriage.' *Blood* Volume 115 pp 4162–7.

Clarke P (2014) *Human Reproduction* Volume 29 (1) pp 184-187.

Human Fertilisation and Embryology Authority. 'Fertility Treatment Options.'

http://www.hfea.gov.uk/fertility-treatment-options-reproductive-immunology.html.

http://www.hfea.gov.uk/docs/FertilityTreatment2012TrendsFigures.PDF.

Love E, Bhattacharya S, Norman C, Smith, Bhattacharya S (2010) 'Research Effect Of Interpregnancy Interval On Outcomes Of Pregnancy After Miscarriage: Retrospective Analysis Of Hospital Episode Statistics In Scotland.' *British Medical Journal* 341: c3967.

Lei L, Spradling A C (2013) 'Female Mice Lack Adult Germ-Line Stem Cells But Sustain Oogenesis Using Stable Primordial Follicles.' *Proceedings of the National Academy of Sciences of the United States of America*, available online at: http://www.pnas.org/content/110/21/8585.

Loh and Makeshuari (2011) cited in Clarke et al (2014) *Human Reproduction* Volume 29 (1) pp 184-187.

Moffett A, Regan L, and Braude P.(2004) 'Natural Killer Cells, Miscarriage and Infertility.' *British Medical Journal* 329 (7477) pp 1283-1285, available online at:

http://www.ncbi.nlm.nih.gov/pmc/articles/PMC534451.

Moffett-King A (2002) 'Natural Killer Cells and Pregnancy.' *Nature Reviews Immunology* 2: pp 656-663

Panzer C, Wise S, Fantini G, Kang D, Munarriz R, Guay A, Goldstein I (2006). 'Impact of Oral Contraceptives on Sex Hormone-Binding Globulin and Androgen Levels: A Retrospective Study in Women with Sexual Dysfunction'. *The Journal of Sexual Medicine* 3 (1): 104-113

Porter T, LaCoursiere Y, Cott J. (2006) 'Immunotherapy for Recurrent Miscarriage.' *Cochrane Database Systematic Review.* 19 (2)

Regan L, Backos M, Rai R (2011) 'The Investigation And Treatment Of Couples With Recurrent First-Trimester And Second-Trimester Miscarriage.' *The Green Top Guideline* 17: pp 1-18.

Royal College of Obstetricians and Gynaecologists (2006) 'Management of Ovarian Hyperstimulation Syndrome.'

Tarozzi N, Bizzaro D, Flamigni C, Borini A (2007) 'Clinical Relevance of Sperm DNA Damage in Assisted Reproduction.' *Reproductive BioMedicine Online* 14(6):746-57.

Tilly J, Johnson J, Canning J, Kaneko T, Pru J (2003) 'Germline Stem Cells and Follicular Renewal in the Postnatal Mammalian Ovary.' *Nature* 428 pp 145-150.

Weimar C, Kavelaars A, Brosens J et al (2012) 'Endometrial Stromal Cells of Women with Recurrent Miscarriage Fail to Discriminate between High- and Low-Quality Human Embryos.' *PLoS One*. Published online 25 July 2012.

ABOUT THE AUTHORS

Claire Chaubert is an experienced professional homeopath and a busy independent midwife. She lives in south east London with her family. Claire has had a broad-ranging career, holding a senior managerial role in central Government before her current work in fertility and midwifery. Claire has a particular interest in helping women recover from previous birth trauma – supporting them through the specialist homeopathic clinic run jointly with Anne Hope, and as an independent midwife. Claire is a member of the Society of Homeopaths (RSHom), registered with the Nursing and Midwifery Council (NMC), a member of the Association of Hypnobirthing Midwives (AHBM), and trained in rebozo technique, maternity reflexology and acupuncture for birthing. Claire is also on the Board of Independent Midwives UK (IMUK). In her spare time she enjoys visiting London's art galleries and museums.

Anne's interest in homeopathy began when homeopathic treatment proved a turning point in her two-year-year old daughter's struggle to recover after contracting meningitis and encephalitis. Although she was initially sceptical, having been brought up using just conventional medicine, observing it work led her to train to become a professional homeopath. In 2003, Anne moved to the West Country and now divides her time running clinics in both London and Devon. She is also a qualified psychologist, has worked as a commercial trainer and a computer programmer, and has taught university courses, including IT, Psychology and Counselling. In addition, she has continued to develop her interest in other alternative health approaches, and practices meditation and yoga. She runs weekend retreat courses in a beautiful setting in Devon, offering a range of programmes in a stress-free setting, for people to experience and learn more about self-empowerment, mindfulness and how to succeed. She also runs introductory courses for those interested in finding out more about crystals, yoga, meditation and the law of attraction.

Printed in Great Britain
by Amazon